CANNABIS
for HEALTH

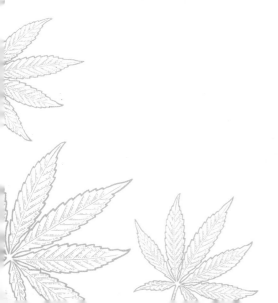

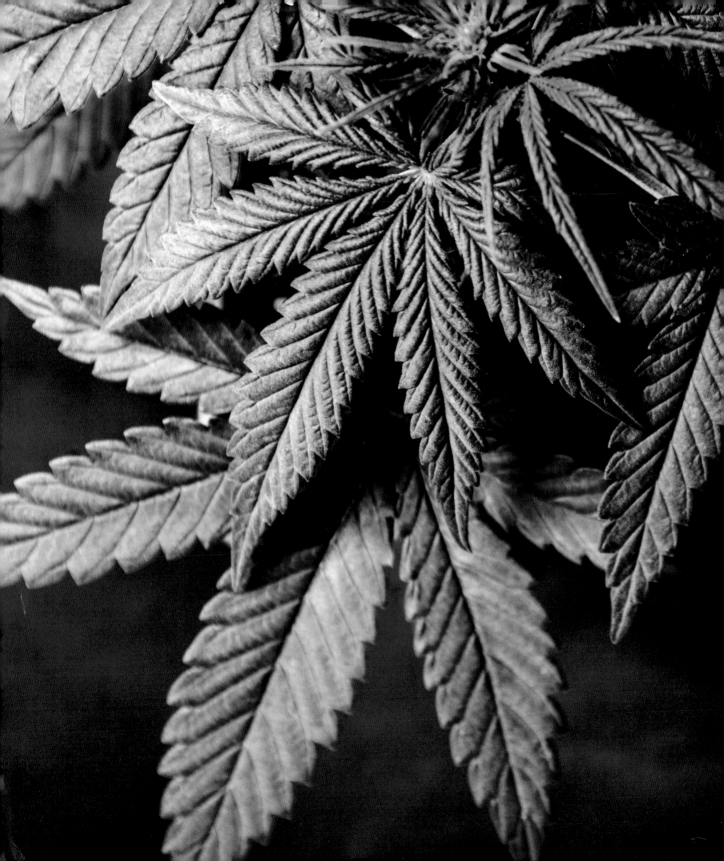

CANNABIS for HEALTH

THE ESSENTIAL GUIDE TO USING CANNABIS FOR TOTAL WELLNESS

Mary Clifton, MD, and Barbara Brownell Grogan

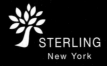

STERLING
New York

STERLING
New York

An Imprint of Sterling Publishing Co., Inc.

ISBN 978-1-4549-4261-0
ISBN 978-1-4549-4276-4 (e-book)

Distributed in Canada by Sterling Publishing Co., Inc.
c/o Canadian Manda Group, 664 Annette Street
Toronto, Ontario M6S 2C8, Canada
Distributed in the United Kingdom by GMC Distribution Services
Castle Place, 166 High Street, Lewes, East Sussex BN7 1XU, England
Distributed in Australia by NewSouth Books
University of New South Wales, Sydney NSW 2052, Australia

For information about custom editions, special sales, and premium and corporate purchases,
please contact Sterling Special Sales at 800-805-5489 or specialsales@sterlingpublishing.com.

Manufactured in Spain

2 4 6 8 10 9 7 5 3 1

sterlingpublishing.com

Cover design by Igor Satanovsky
Interior design by Shannon Nicole Plunkett
Image credits on page 179

CONTENTS

Introduction > *vii*

PART 1: PLANT MAGIC

In Praise of Cannabis > **1**

What Is Cannabis? > **2**

The Endocannabinoid System (ECS) > **3**

PART 2: MAGIC INTO MEDICINE

The Road to Medical Marijuana > **7**

Making Medicine Today > **9**

Legal Questions > **11**

Cannabis and the Workplace > **13**

Testing > 13 — Beating the Test > 14 — Detox and Cleansing Methods > 15

Legalize! > **16**

PART 3: THE LOWDOWN ON THE HEALING HIGH

Body Breakdown: Five Foes > **21**

Getting Back On Track: The Six Pillars of Integrative Nutrition and ECS Tone > **22**

Balanced Diet > 22 — Exercise > 23 — Sleep > 23 — Stress Management > 23

Spirituality > 23 — Socialization > 23

PART 4: THE CANNABIS DISPENSARY

Choosing Products > **25**

Modes of Administration > **26**

Vape Pen > 26 — Flower > 27 — Cannabis Pipe > 28 — Water Pipe > 29

One-Hitter > 30 — Rolling Paper > 30 — Tincture or Edible > 31

PART 5: POWER HEALERS

Cannabis Strains and Their Health Benefits > 33

ACDC > 33 — Chemdawg > 34 — Chernobyl > 34 — Cherry Pie > 34 — Crimea Blue > 34
Crystal Coma > 34 — Death Star > 34 — Dr. Grinspoon > 35 — Durban Poison > 35
Euphoria > 35 — G-13 > 35 — Ghost > 36 — Girl Scout Cookie > 36 — Godfather OG > 36
Grapes > 36 — Harlequin > 36 — Haze > 37 — Headband > 37 — Jack Herer > 37
Kosher Kush > 37 — Lavender > 38 — Mazar > 38 — Medicine Man > 38 — NYC Diesel > 38
OG Kush > 38 — Purple Kush > 39 — Red Congo > 39 — Romulan > 39 — Skunk > 39
Sour Diesel > 39 — Sunset Sherbet > 39 — Tangie > 40 — Trainwreck > 40 — Wedding Cake > 40

PART 6: POWER HEALING WITH CANNABIS

Treatments for 33 Conditions > 43

Accidents > 44 — Addiction and Withdrawal > 46 — ADHD > 49 — ALS > 51 — Anxiety > 53
Autism Spectrum Disorder > 57 — Brain Health > 61 — Cancer > 66 — Depression > 70
Digestive Health > 73 — Elder Care and End of Life > 77 — Epilepsy and Seizures > 80
Eye Health > 85 — Headache > 87 — Heart Health/Heart Disease > 90 — Immune System Health > 93
Inflammation > 96 — Influenza > 98 — Insomnia > 101 — Intimacy and Fertility > 103
Lung Disease > 107 — Lyme Disease > 111 — Metabolic Syndrome > 114 — Multiple Sclerosis (MS) > 117
Pain (Acute and Chronic) > 120 — Parkinson's Disease > 125 — Post-Traumatic Stress Disorder (PTSD) > 128
Psychological Conditions (Bipolar Disorder [Manic Depression] and Schizophrenia) > 131
Skin Conditions > 134 — Stress > 136 — Tics and Tourette Syndrome (TS)/Stuttering > 139
Weight Management > 141 — Women's Health > 145

Glossary > 151

Selected Bibliography > 157

Acknowledgments > 168

About the Authors > 170

Index > 172

Photo Credits > 179

Other Books in the Series > 180

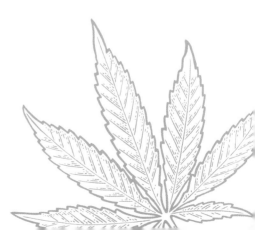

< INTRODUCTION >

CANNABIS: A Medical and Personal Journey

Cannabis has been tied to human history for millennia. Although the plant was first used for fiber and rope in China and on the Indian subcontinent, no one is sure when humanity first discovered the psychoactive properties of cannabis. Archaeologists can date the purposeful burning of cannabis to around 3500 BCE, and it was used in foods in India by 1000 BCE, if not earlier. The ancient Greek historian Herodotus was the first to give textual evidence that cannabis was used in some cultures as a mind-altering substance, around 2000 BCE. The word *cannabis* is probably derived from the Neo-Assyrian and Neo-Babylonian word *qunubu*, meaning "to make smoke."

Psychoactive plants have a long history in human culture. Peyote, or mescaline, has been used by the Indigenous peoples of northern Mexico and the southwestern United States since the beginning of recorded history in North America. Coca leaves were chewed for their stimulatory effects for thousands of years in South America. It has even been proposed that the much-feared berserkers of Viking lore ingested hallucinogenic mushrooms to achieve what has been described as trancelike fury. Consequently, the idea that cannabis may have been part of the human narrative from the very beginning is not hard to accept.

The first documentation of the use of cannabis in Western culture started in the late 1830s in France, when physicians prescribed a number of cannabis-based products to cure a range of frightening ailments and conditions, from consumption (an early name for tuberculosis) and mental illness to plague. At around the same time, a young Irish medical researcher, William Brooke O'Shaughnessy, arrived in India to work as an assistant surgeon for the East India Company. Over the years, O'Shaughnessy conducted significant research in a number of fields, but his most important contribution was the introduction of cannabis as a therapeutic drug to Western medicine. By the latter part of the 19th century and the early 20th century, however, most countries had restricted the use and possession of

< vii >

cannabis and then made it illegal. Criminalizing the possession of cannabis has ultimately led to prison overcrowding in the United States and driven widespread, race-based incarceration of people for even minor infractions of this prohibition.

For centuries, cannabis has been used for spiritual purposes to induce trancelike states in Eastern cultures, as well as a means of treating illness. Ancient cultures attributed various healing properties to cannabis, such as reducing fever, managing nausea and abdominal symptoms, and even treating a stuffy nose. As the 20th century progressed into the 21st, some of those ancient applications began to reemerge. For example, people began to use cannabis to treat the symptoms of nausea and fatigue associated with chemotherapy long before there was a push to legalize cannabis for medical use. At the same time, reports began to surface about the effectiveness of cannabis as a seizure therapy. Current thinking holds that the medicinal properties of cannabis can be effective in treating a variety of medical problems.

Cannabinoid receptors, which are part of the endocannabinoid system (ECS), are scattered

CANNABIS CANNABINOIDS

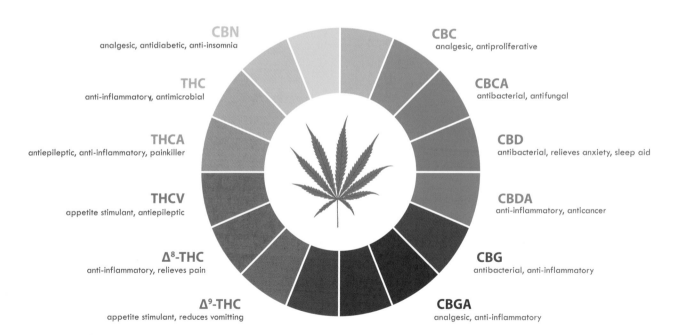

CBN
analgesic, antidiabetic, anti-insomnia

THC
anti-inflammatory, antimicrobial

THCA
antiepileptic, anti-inflammatory, painkiller

THCV
appetite stimulant, antiepileptic

Δ⁸-THC
anti-inflammatory, relieves pain

Δ⁹-THC
appetite stimulant, reduces vomitting

CBC
analgesic, antiproliferative

CBCA
antibacterial, antifungal

CBD
antibacterial, relieves anxiety, sleep aid

CBDA
anti-inflammatory, anticancer

CBG
antibacterial, anti-inflammatory

CBGA
analgesic, anti-inflammatory

throughout the body and impact a wide variety of processes, including pain and stress. Cannabinoids are the active compounds found in cannabis. There are more than 400 cannabinoids, including THC, that react with a number of different receptors in the human body. Cannabinoids sit on those receptors, depending on the type of cannabinoid and the type of receptor. Two receptors are commonly identified—CB1 and CB2—but researchers have also found CB3, CB4, and CB5 receptors in isolated regions of the brain. There are other properties of the cannabis plant that we will explore in this book, including multiple strains of cannabis that have different percentages of cannabinoids and different calming or stimulating effects. Cannabis is now being widely studied and used for the treatment of many health conditions, ranging from anxiety and insomnia to pain management.

As the medical benefits of cannabis have become more established, parts of the United States and other countries around the world have begun to relax legal restrictions and now allow some usage, with proper documentation and medical supervision. Several states in the United States have also begun to allow some recreational use. However, research into cannabis is still regulated by federal law in the United States, which makes experimentation difficult. Nevertheless, much of the social stigma surrounding the use of cannabis has begun to dissipate, and renewed interest in the benefits of cannabis is blossoming.

But that was not the case 35 years ago when my personal journey with cannabis began. I grew up in a small town in northern Michigan in the 1980s. I did well in school, and I think I had a normal childhood with very loving parents, who focused on providing a great education for each of their six kids. In high school, when I wasn't frying my hair with a curling iron and using countless cans of ozone-depleting hairspray, I was experimenting with cannabis, or pot. In my senior year of high school, I unexpectedly became a mother. It was a struggle to put myself through college, and ultimately medical school, as a single mother. Over the years it became clear to me that my early use of cannabis was a method of self-medicating to control my anxieties. In 1985, in small-town northern Michigan, and everywhere else, for that matter, people simply didn't talk about anxiety or other problems like it; instead they self-medicated, typically with alcohol or, in my case, marijuana. Smoking weed made it easier to get through the day, it relieved my anxieties, and it still allowed me to function normally in school and in life.

I stopped using cannabis when I found out about my pregnancy, as well as during the years I spent in college and medical school. At the time, cannabis was frowned upon socially and forbidden professionally. I graduated from medical school with honors and then trained in internal medicine. I was board-certified and then worked in a hospital setting, as well as in my own private practice, for 20 years. During that time, I didn't forget about cannabis, but it didn't enter my mind to use it—I was too busy trying to run a business, raise a family, and conform to the societal norms of the times. I won't say I didn't miss cannabis, but I did avoid it.

Until my brother died.

My brother Tim was a fun-loving and funny man. He spent his entire life in Michigan, working in manufacturing and eventually management. Married and with a family, he was just 52 when he found out that he had colon cancer. It was an aggressive cell type and the cancer advanced quickly, despite the best chemotherapy available. He tried everything and fought the cancer as long as he could, but eventually he was admitted to hospice. I was at his bedside constantly, at the end, trying to manage his care and make him as comfortable as possible. It was hard to control his pain and relieve his anxiety. All the tools of modern medicine were used to help alleviate Tim's pain and every attempt was made to make him comfortable, but none of it was doing the job. I studied his situation and applied everything I knew to try to help him. I would like to say that Tim had a quiet, peaceful death, but that is not the case. I believe he was in pain and experienced skyrocketing anxiety right up to the end, despite the best that modern medicine had to offer.

At about the same time, one of my friends was in a similar situation. Although Fran was suffering from a different type of cancer than my brother's, it also became invasive and ultimately led to her heartbreaking demise. There was a huge difference in her care while she was in hospice, however, because cannabis was available to her as a medication. It helped relieve her pain, attenuate her anxiety, and make her last weeks and months on Earth comfortable and *peaceful*. In short, everything that had been helpful to Fran had been missing from my brother's experience. But I wondered why. Why did the addition of pot, which I had smoked so casually in high school, lead to an end-of-life experience for Fran that was so much better than my brother's? I needed to get an understanding of that experience. What were the mechanics? That search led me to study the scientific literature and learn what science and medicine had to say about cannabis and its effects on the human body and mind. Maybe, just maybe, something wonderful had been right about cannabis all along, and maybe there was something in it that could potentially change the course of medicine in this century.

I began researching all the available scientific literature on cannabis. I talked to people who used it to manage different ailments, to hear what their experiences had been firsthand. What worked and what didn't, as they experimented with different cannabis strains and dosages, routes of administration, timing, and everything else that went into their decision-making.

I talked to experts, I went to conferences, I did everything I could to understand what cannabis is, how it works in the body, and how it can be beneficial for so many people around the world.

I began to produce and shoot short, entertaining, research-packed videos to help people know why and how to use cannabis. Those videos are available to everyone for free at CBDandCannabisInfo.com. I do the research so you don't have to.

I came to the conclusion that my mission as a doctor is to educate people about cannabis, change the minds of those in power, and replace old fallacies about cannabis with new thinking based on science and medical knowledge in order to open up research in the United States and make cannabis available to everyone who needs it. This book is part of that mission. My hope is that the up-to-date information in these pages will help you and many other people around the world understand the science that underpins the beneficial uses of cannabis and also feel confident about using it in your daily life.

Wishing you empowered health,

Mary Clifton, MD

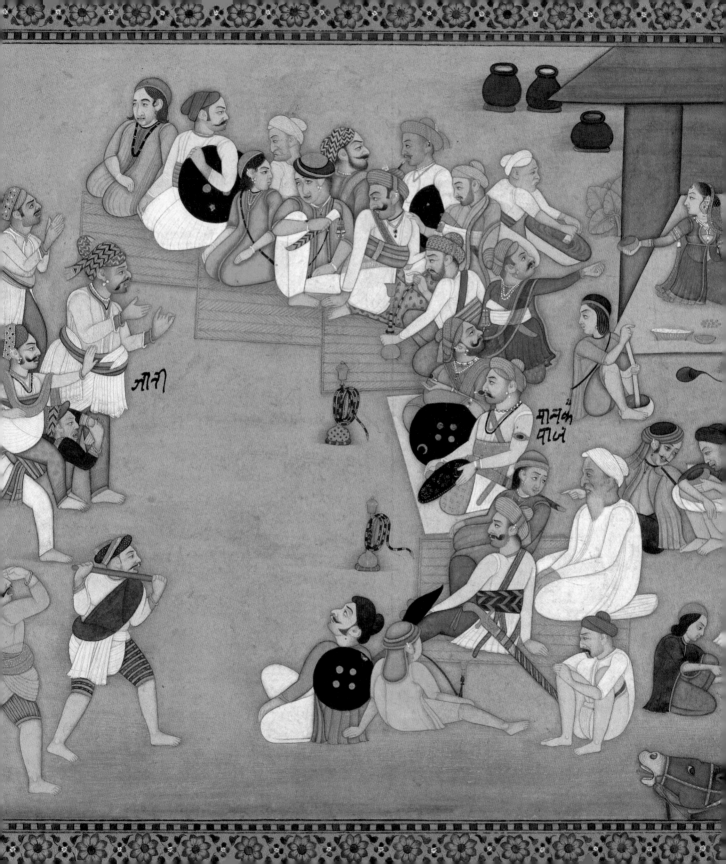

PART 1

< Plant Magic >

IN PRAISE OF CANNABIS

Our fascination with cannabis may be as old as the human story. Shrouded in mysticism, cannabis was used in ancient Eastern cultures for spiritual and bodily well-being; it gradually made its way west to Europe and eventually to colonial America. Early users, like Benjamin Franklin, praised hemp seeds for "abating venereal desires" and touted the leaves as "good against burns." One hundred years later, Robert E. Lee, commander of the Confederate Army during the American Civil War, dreamed of putting cannabis-based "hasheesh" candy into every soldier's pocket to "relieve pain, debility, and fatigue."

The first scientific record of the use of cannabis as medicine was made by physician and chemist William Brooke O'Shaughnessy during his stint with the British East India Company in the 1830s. O'Shaughnessy

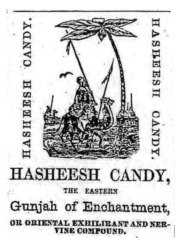

HASHEESH CANDY,

THE EASTERN

Gunjah of Enchantment,

OR ORIENTAL EXHILIRANT AND NER-
VINE COMPOUND.

observed and analyzed how the local population used various parts of the cannabis plant to treat cholera, lung inflammation (or chronic pulmonary obstructive disease [COPD], as it is known today), arthritis, neuralgia, tetanus, seizures, and more. He then conducted his own clinical trials on mice to support his observations and research. O'Shaughnessy's three major books on medicinal plants and his groundbreaking work on the healing powers of cannabis brought East and West together, showcasing ancient Ayurvedic and Persian practices, while laying the scientific groundwork for cannabis as a healer for centuries to come.

It is O'Shaughnessy's legacy that we honor in these pages.

< 1 >

WHAT IS CANNABIS?

Some natural healers, in their reverence for the plant, address cannabis as "her" and "goddess." Botanically speaking, cannabis is a plant like most others, with roots and leaves and flowers. Hemp is the umbrella family name for cannabis, and marijuana (*Cannabis sativa*) is the species name. The two subspecies of cannabis are hemp (*Cannabis sativa sativa*) and recreational marijuana (*Cannabis sativa indica*). For the purpose of this book, we will call every plant in this species "cannabis."

Like many other plants, there are healing compounds in cannabis, such as limonene (which

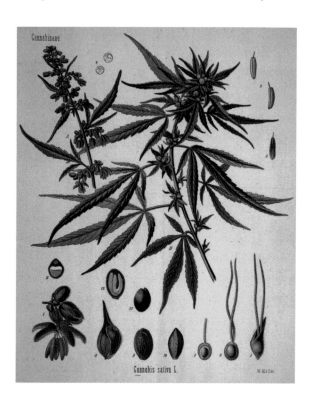

gives lemons their scent) and flavonoids (which make grapes red). Cannabis, however, has an additional set of plant compounds—more than 100 of them, in fact—that other plants don't have. These plant compounds are called cannabinoids, the best known of which are cannabidiol, or CBD, and tetrahydrocannabinol, or THC. While other plant chemicals, like limonene and flavonoids, boost health in various ways—like providing vitamins C or A or protecting cells with their antioxidant power and boosting the immune system—CBD, THC, and other cannabinoids do something even more amazing.

Cannabinoids interact with a system that operates throughout the body that few of us know about. This system helps to regulate our health in countless ways, from processing memories to fighting disease. The positive impact that cannabinoids make on this system is so important that scientists have named it the endocannabinoid system, or ECS (*endo* means "inside"), because it actually produces cannabinoids *inside* the body to keep the system humming along. If the endocannabinoid system stumbles because of an inner upset, such as disease, or an outer upset, such as pollution invading the lungs, then a person can ingest "outer" cannabinoids—such as CBD and THC from the cannabis plant—to help the inner cannabinoids put the endocannabinoid system back on track.

THE ENDOCANNABINOID SYSTEM (ECS)

The endocannabinoid system (ECS) is a complex cell-signaling system involved in a wide variety of processes, including pain, memory, mood, appetite, stress, sleep, metabolism, immune function, and reproductive function. The ECS was identified in the early 1990s by researchers exploring THC, a well-known cannabinoid. Cannabinoids are compounds found in cannabis.

THE ENDOCANNABINOID SYSTEM
HUMAN CANNABINOID RECEPTORS

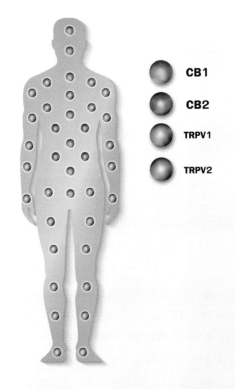

CB1

CB2

TRPV1

TRPV2

All cannabinoids work with the ECS in different ways—but there is one special difference between CBD and THC that can't be denied. Although both CBD and THC can either calm or energize as they heal, THC alone has an intoxicating effect that prompts a high. CBD does not.

The endocannabinoid system is composed of receptors—mainly types called CB1 and CB2—located throughout the body. Endocannabinoids produced by the body interact with ECS receptors to keep bodily functions on course. We can thank researchers from the 1940s for identifying the cannabinoids THC and CBD, and we can thank pioneering Israeli scientist Raphael Mechoulam for his work in the 1980s and '90s identifying the endocannabinoid system and its receptors and how cannabinoids interact with them.

Mechoulam and his team learned that cannabinoids stimulate the CB1 and CB2 receptors to help restore homeostasis and balance in the brain and every other organ in the body where there might be stress or inflammation. With additional research, they were able to show that, when inflammation strikes, the body increases the number of receptors in the inflamed area and produces its own endocannabinoids to interact with them. So, for example, if you were to take a biopsy of an inflamed bowel, you would find higher concentrations of CB receptors and a concentration of endocannabinoids where the body tried to settle down the inflammation.

MANY DIFFERENT STRAINS OF CANNABIS

STRAIN IS USED TO DIFFERENTIATE BETWEEN CANNABIS SATIVA AND INDICA. IT REFERS TO THE SPECIFIC BREED OF EACH INDIVIDUAL PLANT. OVER THE YEARS, FAMILIAL STRAINS HAVE DIVIDED INTO SPECIFIC SUBSECTIONS.

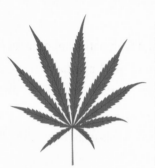

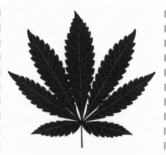

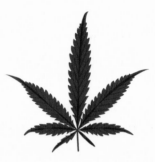

SATIVA STRAINS

Sativa strains have an uplifting effect and offer a cerebral high that includes:

- **Mood elevation**
- **Engaging in in-depth conversations**
- **Thinking creatively**

Sativa strains grow tall and thin—the plant can grow up to 20 feet in an outside garden. Popular strains include:

AMNESIA HAZE
Beloved by morning users, it offers an uplifting boost.

CHERRY AK
With a sweet, fruity smell and taste, this strain can help elevate a bad mood.

GREEN CRACK
Users are rewarded with a blast of exhilarated energy.

SOUR DIESEL
Despite a diesel smell, this strain offers the highest happiness quotient.

INDICA STRAINS

Indica strains have a relaxing, sedative effect, often used to:

- **Reduce stress**
- **Relieve pain**
- **Limit anxiety**

Indica strains are a bushy plant that can grow between 3 and 6 feet tall and are suitable for growing indoors. Popular strains include:

BUBBA KUSH
With a coffee-and-chocolate taste, this strain has a heavy tranquilizing effect.

HEROJUANA
To battle insomnia, this strain induces a heavy, relaxing sleep.

NORTHERN LIGHTS
This pure indica is known to have come from the "mother plant."

SKYWALKER OG
This strain is known for its healing properties for those with PTSD.

HYBRID STRAINS

Hybrid strains offer a mix of effects, combining the traits they inherited from their parent strains. Hybrids are known to:

- **Offer a relaxing body effect**
- **Create balance of mind and body**
- **Limit anxiety**

Of the roughly 779 strains, over half are hybrids. Popular strains include:

BLUE DREAM
Offers a total relaxation while energizing the mind.

GIRL SCOUT COOKIES
This strains a more extrame version of Blue Dream, so go easy!

HEADBAND
Great for pain relief and a feeling of elation.

PINEAPPLE EXPRESS
This sweet, tropical strain leaves one feeling happy and euphoric.

The most prominent endocannabinoids are anandamide and 2-arachidonoylglycerol, or 2-AG. We call them the body's naturally occurring CBD and THC, and you'll hear more about how they interact with receptors to ease conditions later in this book. For example, if you draw fluid from an inflamed knee, you'll find higher concentrations of anandamide in that fluid, showing that endocannabinoids are already working from the inside to restore balance and homeostasis. By ingesting plant, or phyto-, cannabinoids like CBD and THC, you can enhance anandamide's efficiency.

Finally, along with observing naturally occurring endocannabinoids and phytocannabinoids, researchers are producing synthetic (i.e., not plant-derived) cannabinoids from scratch, in laboratories, by replicating cannabinoid molecules.

I have always maintained that whole plants are superior to extracts in both food and medicine; for example, to my mind, vitamin C supplements are less beneficial than eating an orange. I believe the same is true of most synthetic cannabis extracts. In some cases, synthetic concentration of a particularly valuable cannabinoid may boost the ability of the ECS to alleviate serious chronic conditions. Cancer patients or patients with uncontrolled Crohn's disease or ulcerative colitis, for instance, may find that synthetics or distillations offer more arrows in the quiver for treatment. For most cannabis patients, however, optimal benefits to the ECS are obtained from consuming the whole plant.

Sherri Tutkus

Sherri is the founder and CEO of the Green Nurse organization and host of *Green Nurse Radio Show*. Sherri is a cannabis nurse, patient, and advocate who utilizes her 30 years of experience and expert nursing skills as a medical center specialist, clinical nurse liaison, and educator to bridge the gap between patients and the cannabis community. As an educator, she shares her knowledge of the endocannabinoid system and the safe utilization of cannabis with staff at dispensaries, hospitals, clinics, and patients' homes, and she regularly does pop-up events, seminars, and expos. Sherri is an international speaker and has contributed to *Clark's Cannabis: A Handbook for Nurses*, the first cannabis textbook to be published specifically for nurses. It will be available across the United States in 2021.

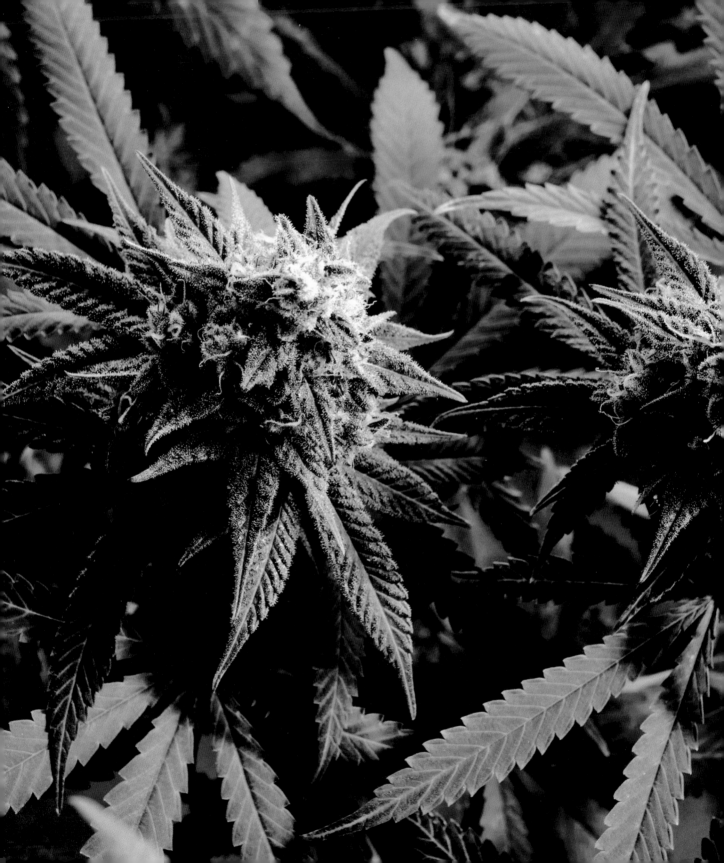

PART 2

< Magic into Medicine >

THE ROAD TO MEDICAL MARIJUANA

Once William Brooke O'Shaughnessy made known his groundbreaking discoveries about the healing properties of cannabis in the mid-1800s, its importance spread like wildfire in the West. By the 1850s it was a prominent entry in the *U.S. Pharmacopeia of Medicines and Dietary Supplements.* For the rest of the 19th century and into the 20th, cannabis was touted as an antidote for myriad upsets and chronic pains, from nausea and fatigue to arthritis and respiratory disease. As an especially effective "nervine," cannabis was even used in the form of a potent hashish candy, which General Lee dispensed to calm his troops. By the turn of the 20th century, the healing power of cannabis was advertised on bottles of Cannabis Americana, in the form of various herbal materials and extracts, and were brought to the marketplace, thanks to a collaboration between pharmaceutical companies Eli Lilly and Company and Parke-Davis & Co. When cannabis was officially criminalized in the United States in the 1930s, production of medicinals stopped, and a dark age for cannabis spread around the world. But while the positive aspects of the plant were given short shrift and the negatives were amplified by the powers that be, brilliant minds were at work under the cover of science.

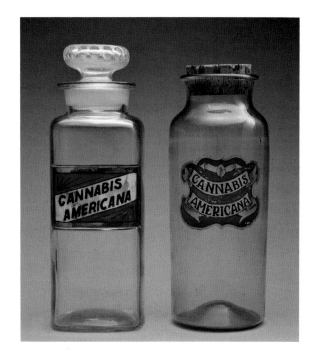

< 7 >

HEMP

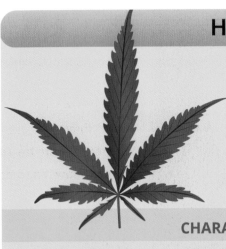

PRODUCT

- CBD oil
- Hemp oil
- Cannabis oil (made from hemp)

CONTAINS

- 0.3% or less of tetrahydrocannabinol (THC)

CHARACTERISTICS

- *Hemp and industry hemp* refer to the cannabis plant strain grown for agricultural products, such as textiles, seeds, and oils.
- The hemp plant is easily grown in most climates and doesn't mind being crowded with other plants; it requires little care.
- Hemp can grow as tall as 20 feet; its leaves are usually bunched near the top of the stem.
- Hemp does not have intoxicating properties.

MARIJUANA

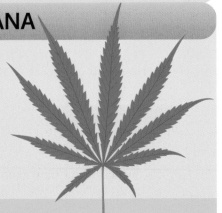

PRODUCT

- THC oil
- Marijuana oil
- Cannabis oil (made from marijuana)

CONTAINS

- 15–20% of tetrahydrocannabinol (THC)

CHARACTERISTICS

- The marijuana plant is known for its flowering tops, which are typically trimmed to encourage higher THC.
- It is shorter than hemp and resembles a bush, with leaves and buds surrounding the main body.
- Growth is carefully monitored and controlled in an isolated, warm, humid area to maximize intoxicating properties; cross-pollination can ruin THC content.
- Marijuana can induce intoxicating side effects.

In 1940, Roger Adams, a researcher in the United States, isolated a chemical compound from the cannabis plant that he called cannabidiol (CBD). Just two years later, in the United Kingdom, a similar compound, tetrahydrocannabinol (THC), was identified, but because of global restrictions on researching cannabis—the pariah of the plant world—little research took place until the 1960s. In that period, visionary Israeli chemist Dr. Raphael Mechoulam and his team, intent on proving the power of cannabis as a healing agent, identified the different chemical structures of CBD and THC. Mechoulam's team discovered that while the structure of THC is linked to inducing a high when ingested, CBD's structure is just different enough not to induce a high. Mechoulam and his colleagues also discovered that, despite their differences, both CBD and THC have the power to heal—and in some cases extraordinarily so. The twin discoveries of how cannabinoids heal and how they work through the endocanna-

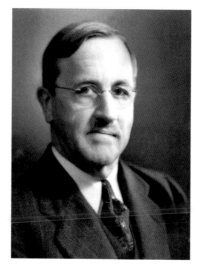

Roger Adams, 1889–1971, scientist who first researched CBD

binoid system were the first of dozens that Mechoulam and others would make over the next 60 years.

In 2013 the door opened further when three-year-old Charlotte Figi stepped onto the world stage, and her compelling story was told on global CNN. Charlotte's parents had watched in helplessness and horror as their child, suffering from a rare form of epilepsy called Dravet syndrome, could barely go an hour without experiencing a seizure. In desperation, they worked with cannabis growers in Colorado to develop a CBD-THC mixture that they named "Charlotte's Web." The product, which immediately calmed and eventually lowered the number of Charlotte's seizures to fewer than four a month, let the world know that cannabis could be respected as a healer. The drug, marketed as Epidiolex®, was not approved by the US Food and Drug Administration for public consumption until 2018. Other research and approvals are ongoing.

MAKING MEDICINE TODAY

The future of cannabis in medicine probably lies in Israel. For decades, the forefront of cannabis research has been centered in Tel Aviv because of pioneer researcher Raphael Mechoulam. Not only did he discover the chemical structure and interaction of THC and CBD with the ECS, but he also became the first researcher to state that CBD might be an effective treatment for seizure disorder.

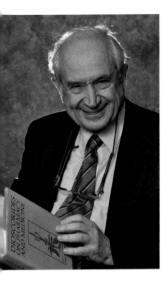

Israeli organic chemist and professor of medicinal chemistry at the Hebrew University of Jerusalem, Raphael Mechoulam (b. 1930)

Because of Mechoulam's work, research blossomed in Tel Aviv; the latest innovation is a synthetic, stable cannabiodiolic acid (CBDA) molecule. This molecule is also pure, meaning that there are no residual impurities that may have been introduced when retrieving the CBDA from the plant itself. These acids, in their natural form, break down easily before delivering their benefits. That is why cannabis has been heated or burned for centuries. That process, called decarboxylation, transforms the cannabinoid molecule into its active form, allowing it to have an optimal healing effect. Still, new research suggests that the original carboxylated form, CBDA and THCA, may have medicinal properties as well.

Decarboxylation is important because it's possible that cannabiodiolic acid, the stable precursor molecule to CBD before decarboxylation, may be a more effective treatment for depression, and possibly for nausea, than CBD products. Why? Most likely because cannabiodiolic acid is active in the ECS pathways that affect serotonin, the neurotransmitter. Although it makes us feel good and eases depression, serotonin can also prompt nausea in order to oust toxins from the body.

CBDA helps optimize serotonin to ease depression and, working with the HT-5 ECS receptor, CBDA helps thwart serotonin release in order to limit nausea. This research is preliminary, as of this writing, but promising because it could be a potential breakthrough in handling several common diseases.

CBDA, as it turns out, might be even more versatile than current research suggests. CBDA does not bind to the main cannabinoid receptors CB1 and CB2, as CBD does. Instead, it interacts directly with the ECS in other ways, partly by inhibiting the release of cyclooxygenase-2, which prompts inflammation and pain. Celebrex® and other nonsteroidal anti-inflammatory medications (NSAIDs) work this way. In fact, the chemical structure of CBDA and some NSAIDs are similar.

Another phytocannabinoid showing promise is cannabichromene (CBC). CBC is a by-product of the breakdown of cannabichromene carboxylic acid when exposed to a heat source. It doesn't bind well to CB1 and CB2 receptors, so it doesn't

Cannabidiolic Acid
(CBDA)

Cannabidiol
(CBD)

have the same effects; that is, it doesn't produce a high. However, it does bind to other ECS receptors, including receptors that help mitigate the sensation of pain.

CBC may also contribute to the "entourage effect"—the cumulative benefit of multiple cannabinoids working together to modulate the response of cannabis in the body for optimal healing. Products that include multiple cannabinoids, such as CBD, THC, and CBC, as well as other chemicals such as terpenes and flavonoids, are referred to as "full spectrum" and are often preferred to an isolate product, which has a single-focus cannabinoid. While an isolate is sometimes preferred for treating specific conditions within a discrete time period, it does not deliver the general and long-standing well-being that comes with a multifaceted product.

CBC on its own may have beneficial effects in areas beyond pain management. For example, one of the anti-inflammatory properties of CBC causes an increased expression of another cannabinoid, anandamide. Often called the bliss molecule, anandamide plays a role in the feeding and

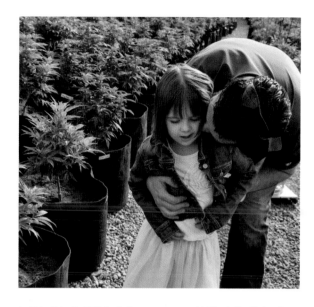

In this Feb. 7, 2014 photo, seven-year-old Charlotte Figi, whose parents describe her as once being severely and untreatably ill, walks inside a greenhouse housing a special strain of medical marijuana known as Charlotte's Web, which was named after Charlotte early in her treatment, at a grow location in a remote spot in the mountains west of Colorado Springs.

reward pathways of the brain, as well as in pain management. (The bliss molecule is also present in chocolate, which may explain a lot!) Data suggests that increased release of anandamide may play a role in fighting breast cancer, but there is not yet enough data to support that claim.

LEGAL QUESTIONS

The story of cannabis as an illicit drug in America is a long and confounding one, in which cannabis was once king of medicines and then relegated to the lowest rank as a dangerous and subversive substance. Now cannabis is slowly and surely

making its way back up the ladder to reverence, rung by rung.

In the early years of the 20th century, cannabis was known to bring relief from anxiety during wartime; dull the pain of the sick and dying; and bring focus, clarity, and calm to those suffering from depression and psychiatric trauma. Things started to change around 1900, however, beginning with the influx of Mexican immigrants into the United States. When it became commonly known that some immigrants smoked marijuana, the existing prejudice against Mexicans was further stoked into racist hysteria over the effects of the drug among its users, presumably violence and crime, as well as other social ills. A similar narrative played out in the 1920s and 1930s with African American artists like legendary jazz musician Louis Armstrong, who was known to enjoy smoking cannabis as a conduit for musical experimentation and creativity. But while Armstrong and others were creating an art form that would influence American culture for decades, politicians and policy makers set about demonizing cannabis and jazz as satanic. And that is why, in a nutshell, cannabis became illegal in the United States. In the 1930s Harry Anslinger, director of the newly founded Federal Bureau of Narcotics and a rabid nationalist and white supremacist, told Americans that cannabis use by immigrants and African Americans was promoting debauchery and sowing fear across the nation. He placed cannabis in all its forms on a list of illicit

substances called Schedule I drugs. The penalty for possessing any of them was incarceration. Cannabis remains on the list of Schedule I drugs to this day.

Here's the good news: As evidence of the healing power of cannabis continues to mount, its reputation is moving up the ladder of medical acceptability as well. As of June 2018, the FDA has approved Epidiolex®, a high-THC pharmaceutical, for the treatment of two rare forms of epilepsy. Also, as of 2018, some 30 states in the United States have legalized marijuana for medical use, meaning formulations can be purchased if they're prescribed and if the patient has a medical marijuana card.

In addition, several states, as well as Washington, DC, now allow residents over the age of 21 to grow a limited number of THC-rich cannabis plants for recreational use. Growing CBD-rich, low-THC cannabis, often called hemp, is legal in all 50 states thanks to the Farm Bill of December

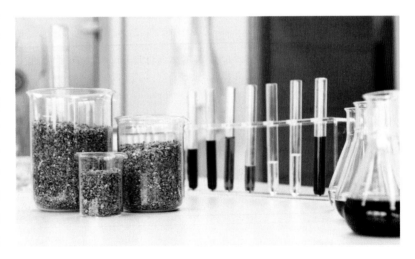

2018. But there are restrictions. The bill does not fully lift hemp's Schedule I status, so growers need approved licensing, and hemp products created under strict regulations can cross state lines only when transported by the approved producer.

Still, even as cannabis becomes more mainstream, patients and recreational users need to be aware of the legal challenges they may face in society, the workplace, and beyond.

CANNABIS AND THE WORKPLACE

Testing

With so many concerns about the legal complexities surrounding the use of cannabis, both recreationally and medicinally, people are worried, understandably, about the security of their jobs. At the same time, employers worry about setting up logical and reasonable policies regarding the use of cannabis, in its various formulations, among employees.

Now, more than ever, people are reaching for cannabinoids for medical and recreational use, as the legal status of cannabis products continues to change and as it becomes clearer that safety concerns surrounding their use are likely exaggerated. As it turns out, those previously questionable products are in fact safe and effective for the treatment of a number of different conditions. Now we need to figure out the most accurate way for employers to test employees, if there are any concerns about safety in the workplace resulting from employees' use of cannabis for either recreational or health purposes.

Currently when companies test employees, they look for a specified level of hydroxylated THC, acquired from the cannabinoid formulation that an employee may have consumed. THC is the intoxicating ingredient in the cannabis plant that creates a high when cannabinoid formulations are consumed. Afterward, THC metabolizes in the body and is stored in fat as THC-COOH, or tetrahydrocannabinol carboxylic acid. This metabolite (the end product of metabolism) is then measured in a laboratory, with a cutoff of 50 nanograms per milliliter, which is where a test turns positive. Some companies have a zero-tolerance policy and terminate employees whose test results show any identifiable level of THC. Different regulatory agencies manage the testing—and there's plenty of data surrounding the test—to make sure that it's done properly. In fact, it's very difficult to get a false positive. That wasn't the case early on, when taking a drug like ibuprofen (Motrin® or Advil®) could lead to a false positive, but that risk has been cleared up for some time now. It's safe to say that there's really nothing that can contribute to the development of a false positive test.

The great thing about CBD in most CBD formulations is that the THC concentration in the formulations is so low. That concentration should be tested, measured, and not sold by the manufacturer if the THC level is higher than 0.3 percent. Consequently, you would have to ingest about 2,000 milligrams of CBD full-spectrum formulations every day to potentially test positive on a drug test. However, it is possible that an unscrupulous CBD company might allow a batch of CBD to leave the factory with a higher concentration of THC, which could subsequently lead to problems for the consumer. If you have any concerns about the quality of a CBD product, the best choice—so as not to get any THC at all—is to use a CBD isolate rather than a full-spectrum or broad-spectrum product.

Beating the Test

The half-life of THC and other cannabinoids is about 20 hours, and it takes between five and six half-lives to completely remove a drug from your system. That means that it'll take somewhere between five and eight days for a single dose to be fully out of your body's system. That process, however, can be affected by BMI (body mass index) because cannabinoids are lipophilic molecules. Cannabinoids are readily absorbed into fats,

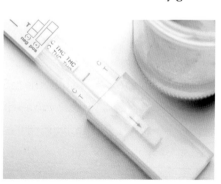

so a higher BMI will definitely put you at a disadvantage. And don't think that exercise will help, either. A high level of exercise may actually mobilize the metabolites from fat stores and raise the level of carboxylated THC in your bloodstream.

Hair testing is a different story. Daily use of THC and other cannabinoids can show up in your hair for about three months, but hair testing for irregular use is unreliable. Most companies rely on urine testing for their employees.

If you are wondering if it is possible to beat a drug test, the answer is this: No particular method of beating a drug test is going to be 100 percent foolproof.

It is important to bear in mind that if your employer is testing you for THC, the company is probably doing so to keep your workplace safe for you and your fellow workers, as well as to ensure the safety of the consumer who buys the products you make. Intoxication in the workplace cannot be tolerated. There's a zero-tolerance policy on the roadways for intoxication, and there's a zero-tolerance policy in most workplaces for the same very good reason.

Drug tests look specifically for the THC metabolite—the end product that is present in urine after your body breaks down the THC. It's called carboxylated THC-COOH, and these drug tests are very sensitive to that particular metabolite. There is a potential for false positives at roadside testing, however, because it is targeted at consumption, which could have occurred anytime in the recent past, but does not measure acute intoxication or recent use. Undoubtedly, there will be some legal issues surrounding exactly how roadside testing for cannabinoid formulations is going to play out on a broader level. Whether or not the results of the testing will stand up in court remains to be seen.

Detox and Cleansing Methods

Multiple mechanisms have been suggested for the best means of detoxing and cleaning out your system. The most common method involves aggressive hydration—drinking a ton of water—and then taking B_{12} vitamins to make your urine turn yellow. If you drink a lot of water without taking B_{12}, however, your urine is going to look more like water than urine and won't pass any type of drug test. It will be rejected if it looks as though you've tampered with it. On the other hand, taking B_{12} in tandem with aggressive hydration will often decrease the THC concentration in urine without changing its usual yellow appearance too much, so the drug test can go through. With a lower percentage of THC metabolites in the urine, you might be able to squeak by a drug test.

A lot of herbal teas and detox cleansers might seem to work over the course of several days to weeks, with discontinued consumption of whatever cannabis formulation you've been using, but at that point the level of THC in your system would have come down naturally. So, in all likelihood, your own body is doing an equally effective job of detoxing your system as any herbal tea or other cleanser.

Again, none of the detox products, plans, or protocols that you may find online are 100 percent foolproof, and please don't even consider contaminating your urine specimen with products like Visine®, bleach, salts, or detergents. It won't do you any good. All those products are readily identifiable by testing companies.

According to the Mayo Clinic testing website, you should be able to pass a drug test in just three days after a single use of a cannabis product, but if you're consuming that product four times a week, it may take five to eight days for your body to clear out all the metabolites. If you're consuming on a daily basis, you'll need to spend at least ten days in detoxification to clear your system for drug testing; chronic daily consumption may take up to a month of detoxification.

Please don't forget that, in a lot of cases, sobriety is a job requirement, particularly in areas like transportation and manufacturing, where your safety, the safety of your coworkers, and, ultimately, the safety of the consumer will be in danger if you are intoxicated on the job. The best way to avoid that calamity (not just failing a drug test) is to avoid using drugs that will show up on the test in the first place.

Unlike drug testing for the THC metabolite, the picture for CBD is considerably brighter. That's because CBD has no intoxicating effect. It won't get you high or in any way dull your capacity to respond effectively and safely in a setting where intoxication would be a liability, so there is no risk of impairment or any danger, as a result, to yourself and others. But just to be on the safe side, if you know you'll be given a drug test, please consider using a pure CBD, known as CBD isolate, so there won't be even a trace of THC in your system. If you are taking a CBD product for health reasons, let your human resources department know. They can partner with you to help make the very best decisions about managing your health care.

LEGALIZE!

Millions of people across the United States and around the world use cannabinoid formulations that appear to be less harmful than alcohol, according to most studies, and certainly less harmful than many other products that lead to intoxication. Cannabis usage is occurring across the population, regardless of socioeconomic status, age, gender, or race. Population studies in New York State, as well as in Canada and other countries, repeatedly reveal that about 17 percent of residents have used cannabis in the preceding year. Even though Black and brown people are responsible for only half of the cannabis that is used or distributed, the overwhelming majority of legal ramifications for the possession or use of cannabis is borne by those populations.

To date, a majority of states and the District of Columbia in the United States have legalized cannabis usage medically (36) or recreationally (15), and federal legalization seems a real possibility in the near future. However, licenses for sales of

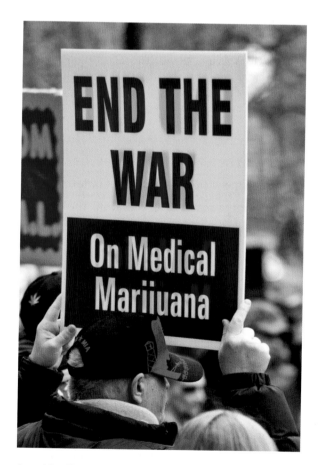

An unidentified protester holds up at sign at the 40th annual Hash Bash at the University of Michigan campus on Saturday, April 2, 2011, in Ann Arbor, Michigan. Several thousand people attended the event.

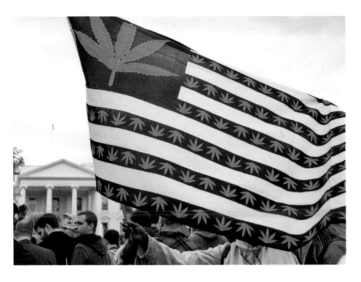

Protesters rally in support of the legalization of marijuana in front of the White House in Washington, DC, on April 2, 2016

medical marijuana have overwhelmingly gone to wealthy white men who have no criminal record. As a result, the medical cannabis industry in the United States may be perpetuating the harm of the war on drugs and its ongoing impact on Black and brown communities.

In many states where cannabis is currently illegal, a resident can buy cannabis legally, right across the border, in another state. However, upon return, that person may be imprisoned, often for an extended period, for a product that was legally purchased over the state line. Fortunately, that sad reality has moved a number of states to decriminalize medical marijuana, as well as to expunge the criminal records of some people arrested previously for possessing small amounts of cannabis. Most states, however, have taken only minor steps to help communities that

continue to be targeted by unfair drug law enforcement.

As the United States moves toward broader legalization patterns, state by state, any cannabinoid formulation with a level of THC greater than 0.3 percent is prohibited for any purpose by the federal government. However, CBD produced with low levels of THC is legal in all 50 states. At the same time, other countries continue to have more severe penalties than those in the United States. In some Asian, African, and Middle Eastern countries, possession of even small amounts of cannabis is punishable by imprisonment for several years. By contrast, countries such as Canada, Georgia (in Eastern Europe), South Africa, and Uruguay have legalized recreational cannabis, and in Spain and the Netherlands there are policies that allow licensed establishments to sell cannabis.

The use of medical cannabis has been legalized in Argentina, Australia, Canada, Chile, Colombia, Croatia, Cyprus, Germany, Greece, Israel, Italy, Jamaica, Lithuania, Luxembourg, Macedonia, Norway, the Netherlands, New Zealand, Peru, Portugal, Poland, Switzerland, and Thailand. Other countries allow restricted sales of certain high-THC cannabinoid formulations that are synthetically manufactured by pharmaceutical companies, such as Sativex®, Marinol®, and Epidiolex®.

Why should we legalize cannabis? There are so many good reasons to proceed with legalization that it's hard to understand why we haven't moved more quickly to make it a reality. These are the biggest reasons for legalization:

- **HARM REDUCTION.** The criminalization of cannabis disproportionately harms brown and Black people and leads to tremendous violence and disruption in their communities. Laws have not been effective in curbing young people's access to cannabis, and when law enforcement officers get involved and incarceration takes place, the welfare of both the individual and their entire family is at risk. Not only do members of the family lose the ability to interact and share their lives with the incarcerated individual, they also lose potential income for the family and spend a shocking amount of money on bail and legal fees. The prison system has spawned a network of other industries that work together to extract inordinate sums of money from families who will do anything to protect their loved ones in these circumstances. For some individuals, possession of small amounts of cannabis has led to sentences that have stretched out for decades.

- **JOB CREATION/ECONOMIC OPPORTUNITY.** With legalization of cannabis, one of the nation's largest cash crops would be regulated, creating a formal economy instead of a secondary market, which, in turn, would result in economic opportunities for people at nearly every level of the cannabis industry. If you have an interest in cannabis, there is a role for you in this emerging industry.

- **COST SAVINGS.** State and local governments would acquire significant new sources of tax revenue with legal regulation of marijuana sales. Tax revenue could be used to revitalize neighborhoods that have been—and continue to be—negatively impacted by the war on drugs, by supporting early childhood education and rebuilding crumbling infrastructure. If cannabis criminal records were expunged, resources currently being used to ensure public safety and manage correctional facilities and the courts could be released to pay for more pressing projects in high-risk communities.

- **CUSTOMER SAFETY.** Effective and reliable product testing could be standardized across legitimate cannabis markets. Consequently, consumers would be better informed about the products they chose to buy. The production of cannabis formulations could be monitored from seed to sale, with more safety and reliability than almost any other consumable product on the market today. Customers could rely on strong product testing as well, to avoid contaminants such as heavy metals in soil that could be absorbed by and concentrated in hemp plants.

Despite the expense and extreme punitive measures in place, the war on drugs has not protected American children from experimenting with cannabis. Further product regulation and labeling could be enforced in a legalized environment to ensure that young people are not targeted as customers by the industry.

We can't overstate the significance of criminal justice reform and the necessity to end institutional racism in America, much of which has been built on the war on drugs and has disproportionately targeted and ruined the lives of millions of Black and brown people. African Americans are nearly four times as likely as white Americans to be arrested for cannabis possession, even though cannabis is used at roughly the same rate across the country, regardless of skin color. It's time to recognize that the criminalization of marijuana has been a failure. It's time for legalization, with regulation that ensures revenue from sales is reinvested in communities hit hardest by the war on drugs.

Even 10 years ago, a conversation about federal legalization of marijuana would have been considered too "radical," but today we are beginning to see sweeping changes in the way cannabis is perceived by our society. Those changes are supported by scientific data and a record of at least 4,000 years of human experience with both the recreational and health benefits of using cannabis in various forms.

David L. Nathan

Cannabis advocate David L. Nathan, MD, DFAPA, a Princeton, New Jersey–based psychiatrist, writer, speaker, educator, and consultant, is also the founder and board president of Doctors for Cannabis Regulation. Dr. Nathan is a founding steering committee member of New Jersey United for Marijuana Reform, which was launched in early 2015, the same year he became the first physician in New Jersey history to testify in favor of cannabis legalization before the state legislature. In 2019, Dr. Nathan was one of two physicians to testify at the first US House Judiciary Committee hearing on cannabis legalization. He coauthored a landmark article on cannabis regulation with former US surgeon general Joycelyn Elders for the *American Journal of Public Health*. He has advocated for cannabis legalization in major news outlets, including CNN, *The New York Times*, *The Wall Street Journal*, the *San Francisco Chronicle*, and *Politico*. Currently, he is the chief medical advisor for 4Front Ventures, a multistate medical cannabis company.

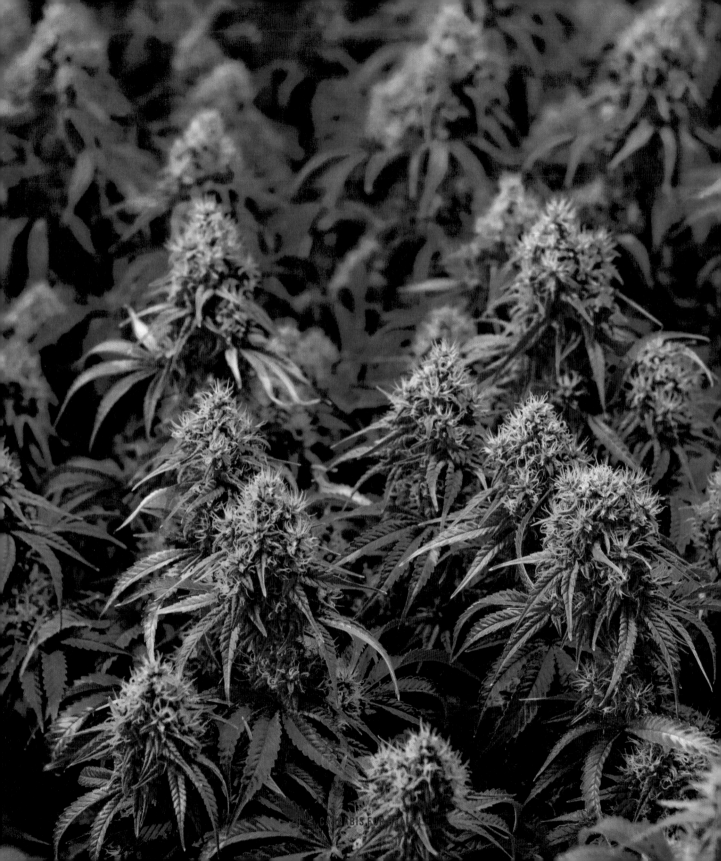

PART 3

< The Lowdown on the Healing High >

BODY BREAKDOWN: Five Foes

How do ailing bodies mend? In order to understand how cannabis helps us right a sinking ship, it's important to recognize symptoms of five foes that are the root of most illnesses. We'll introduce them here, but you'll have an opportunity to learn more about them in part 6, "Power Healing with Cannabis: Treatments for 33 Conditions." This unwelcome team of health foes stealthily infiltrates and breaks down your system. When you realize you've been invaded, you could be facing a crisis. But know this: It is never too late to foil an attack.

1. **INFLAMMATION.** While a little inflammation is integral to healing—think of the puffy red area that forms around a healing cut—a lot of inflammation over a long period leads to a system breakdown. Inflammation can cause a number of serious conditions, ranging from arthritis to cancer.

2. **STRESS.** Like inflammation, stress can save your life, sharpening your senses and raising your reaction time to cope with dire situations. But too much stress causes overload in every organ of the body. It also aggravates existing or dormant underlying ailments that are just waiting for a trigger.

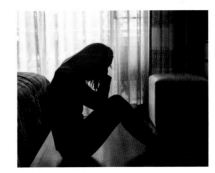

3. **SLEEP DEPRIVATION.** We need sleep to think clearly, improve memory, solve problems, face the day with optimism, and heal. Sleep gives us time to reboot—and we need a full seven to eight hours every night. Without that healing, strengthening time, we are more vulnerable to accidents, infections, depression, and even high blood pressure.

< 21 >

4. **ANXIETY.** The result of continual stress, anxiety lies dormant, quietly building as you endure a demanding or unhappy relationship or job, until it suddenly pounces—possibly in the form of a panic attack with chest pain and heart palpitations. Unaddressed, anxiety attacks can become chronic, returning again and again without notice, leading to or complicating other physical and psychological disorders.

5. **DEPRESSION.** Whether triggered by a tragic event, such as the loss of a spouse or a child, or the result of a long-standing illness, depression is more than a period of feeling blue. Over time this condition can lead to fatal high blood pressure, heart disease, stroke, and suicide.

GETTING BACK ON TRACK: The Six Pillars of Integrative Nutrition and ECS Tone

While CBD and medical marijuana can go a long way toward fighting the foes of our well-being, they can only go so far. They must be part of integrative nutrition, a bigger, more inclusive, healing lifestyle. Essentially, integrative nutrition is a practice that combines six healing lifestyle practices—pillars that boost all-around, high-functioning body and spirit—which in turn lead to a "toned" ECS (endocannabinoid system). When your body's ECS is toned, it is strong and runs smoothly, as a result of basic good health.

When it falters, it can quickly return to optimal function with outside input from the six pillars of integrative nutrition, together with a boost from healing cannabis.

You may have built up some of the six pillars of integrative nutrition over years, perhaps as you've made a daily practice of nurturing your family relationships and spiritual connections. Even if you've neglected other important practices, such as healthy diet and exercise, you can start to build them up now.

1. **BALANCED DIET.** Foods rich in omega-3 fatty acids, including olive oil, nuts, avocados, green leafy vegetables, and high-fat fish, like salmon, support the ECS. Avoid processed foods, which work to lower endocannabinoid production, disrupt the ECS, and set the stage for diabetes, heart disease, and other chronic ailments. Studies show that probiotics, such as yogurt and sauerkraut, increase the response of cannabinoid receptors in the intestines, promoting healthy gut function.

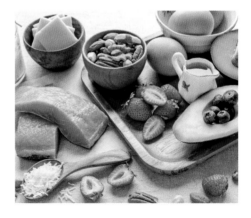

2. **EXERCISE.** Scientists have recognized this mighty medicine as a 20th-century wonder drug for its extraordinary capacity to heal and maintain wellness. Studies show that increased movement boosts cannabinoid receptors and their interaction with endocannabinoids in the brain and throughout the body, increasing mental sharpness, well-being, and more.

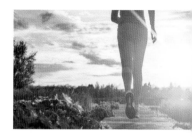

3. **SLEEP.** Quality sleep is a natural reset button. Research shows that it makes us more alert, wards off inflammation and pain, and helps manage stress and maintain optimal weight—actions also regulated by a healthy ECS. Scientists have found that certain endocannabinoids can increase in number at night and that certain receptors are more responsive to them. Sleep boosts a healthy ECS, and, in a positive synergy, a healthy ECS boosts sleep.

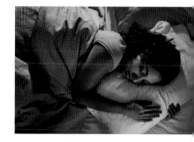

4. **STRESS MANAGEMENT.** A 2016 NIH (National Institutes of Health) study reported that chronic stress decreases the production of ECS receptors and endocannabinoids, lowering the ECS response to inflammation, compromising immune function, and setting the stage for anxiety, chronic pain, memory loss, and other unwelcome health conditions. Reassess your lifestyle and calm down.

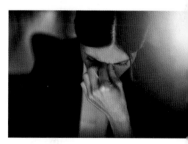

5. **SPIRITUALITY.** Whether you pray to a higher power or practice meditation, chanting, or yoga, experts say these activities evoke a relaxation response, promoting mental and physical well-being. Such practices may help the ECS remain balanced, warding off stress and the diseases it can trigger.

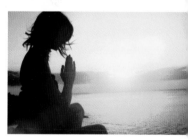

6. **SOCIALIZATION.** Similar to spirituality, socializing with others brings us a sense of community, the understanding that we are not alone. Relationships with friends, family, a beloved partner—preferably all of them—are key. Decades of research show that giving and receiving increases the chemical oxytocin, the release of which reinforces trust and empathy and helps minimize stress, anxiety, depression, and pain while encouraging an optimal heart rate. All those factors help the ECS maintain balance.

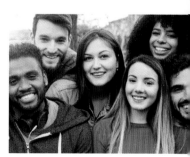

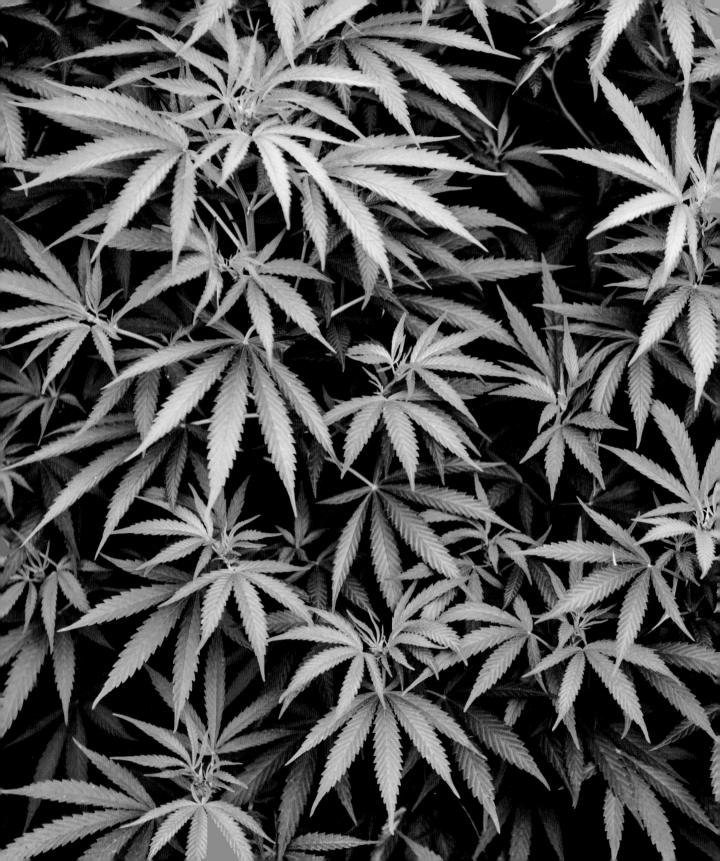

PART 4

< The Cannabis Dispensary >

CHOOSING PRODUCTS

Whether you're purchasing a cannabis product for the first time or have been supplied with them through other channels for decades, the amazing selection of cannabis products in legal dispensaries—and the lack of anxiety in choosing them—is becoming a way of life in America. Now that medical-use cannabis is allowed in more than half the United States, and since even more states have decriminalized possession, the new menus available at legal dispensaries can be overwhelming. It's like trying to choose a dish from the menu at your favorite fabulous (but expensive!) restaurant during Restaurant Week. So many options! Such great deals! Who thought of this recipe? What on Earth is in that reduction?

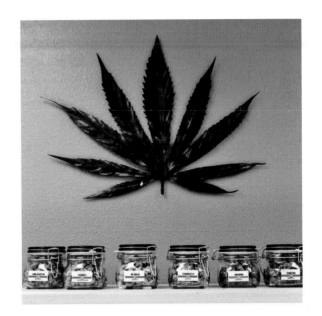

As a first-timer considering cannabis therapy, here are some basics to keep in mind before you purchase a cannabis product:

- Always read up on your local laws before going to the dispensary.

- Always carefully read the label on any cannabis product and look for the following information:

  » The percentage of THC. A maximum of 0.3 percent THC comprises a legal product across the United States.

< 25 >

» The type of product, depending on your needs. Is it full spectrum, broad spectrum, or isolate?

» Plant origin. Products made from plants produced by certified organic growers in the United States are the purest because US agricultural rules are so stringent.

» Third-party testing. Be sure that the manufacturer has sent the product to a third-party laboratory for objective testing to ensure there is no trace of contamination.

Finally, consider which mode of administration is optimal for you.

MODES OF ADMINISTRATION

Vape Pen

Vape pens are efficient delivery systems for weed oil. The oil is extracted from the marijuana plant and then mixed with what is considered a harmless vehicle, such as certain oils or sugars, so that the formulation is thin enough to be used in vaporizing cartridges. Usually this oil is a coconut or vegetable oil, but products like polyethylene glycol and glycerin are sometimes added to sweeten the smoke. Chemicals also give the smoke a very white, thick appearance when exhaled. Flavorings that are sometimes found in tobacco or cannabis vaporizers are thought to have contributed to a surge in lung disease recently. The safety of vaporizers continues to be studied, and it's likely that commonly used products in vaporizers will be restricted or regulated in the future. For some, the safety of these vaporizers continues to be a real concern.

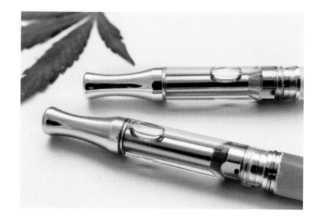

Vaporized cannabis is especially valuable when you want to be discreet about smoking in a social gathering or any other place where the odor or appearance of a pipe or marijuana cigarette could be considered obtrusive. A cannabis vaporizer is elegant and difficult to differentiate from a tobacco vaporizing pen. However, it's important to choose a vaporizer that allows you to buy replacement cartridges, rather than buying a single-use vaporizer that you toss into the garbage after the cartridge is used. Vaporizers are available in many forms, potencies, and sizes.

It should be noted that it's not legal to use a cannabis vaporizer anyplace where it's not legal to use cannabis in cigarette form. But that doesn't stop people from using vaporizers in restaurants, while walking down the street, or in other public venues.

Personal-use vaporizers that use whole-flower cannabis are especially appealing. These products have a small oven that superheats the cannabis without igniting it, in a process that gives the user the benefits of the cannabinoids and terpenes in the flower, while decreasing exposure to carcinogens by 90 percent (according to studies). Due to the superheating process, the taste of cannabis is often less herbal and sweeter, and the heavy, lingering odor of the smoke is not as pronounced compared to cannabis cigarettes. So gadgets like these offer a nice alternative for a cannabis user who wants to keep private things private.

Flower

Flower is simply a new name for old-fashioned cannabis in its usual form, also known as bud or weed. Flower is still the standard for most dispensaries, where you'll often find a menu with a number of options that describe the effects of a particular strain, as well as a selection of popular strains that are available in cigarettes, known as pre-rolls.

There are many attributes to consider when choosing the strain that's best for you. Be sure that the product smells fresh, with hints of the terpenes you are looking for, such as a scent of lemon, a mild scent of diesel, or a sweetness without any staleness or hint of mold or mildew. Remember that a dispensary is a business, and a product that may be on sale or initially offered might be one that the dispensary owner wants to move—not because it's the best product for your particular condition. Each individual flower should be carefully trimmed of stray leaves and should have a soft, spongy feel when handled; any cracking, breaking, or excessive dryness could suggest a dated product. Proper trimming is paramount to the development of an ideal bud, allowing the flower to be perfectly framed. If you are selecting a top-shelf cannabis that appears leafy instead of closely trimmed, it's likely the sugar leaves surrounding the bud were considered too precious to trim and throw away because

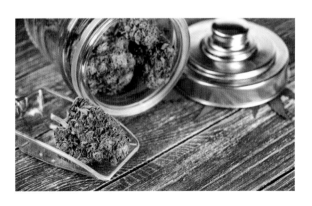

they are covered with the tiny, hairlike trichomes rich in THC and other cannabinoids as well as the terpenes and flavonoids you're looking for.

Improperly cared-for cannabis has a tendency to have high levels of cannabinol (CBN), a by-product of degradation. Stems and seeds should be minimal or nonexistent; low-quality products tend to be light, leafy, and wispy. Excessive heat or underwatering may limit development of trichomes—the hairlike protrusions on the flowers that produce concentrated cannabinoids, especially THC and other plant chemicals. Improper storage may also contribute to this problem.

By contrast, the highest-quality cannabis, the top-shelf buds, will stand out in a sea of green. A highly diverse color spectrum and complex aromas will make it clear that you're looking at the best of the best. Depending on where you live, these first-class cannabis strains can come with an extremely high price tag. They will likely have a thick coat of sugary resin, containing the high concentrations of cannabinoids and terpenes that have powerful effects. Under the best growing conditions, the buds will be not only dense but also chunky, especially if the grower has used advanced carbon dioxide levels during particular parts of the growth cycle, as well as other innovative growing techniques that enhance the production of THC in the plant. The finest herb should be truly sticky from a resin-rich frosting of trichomes but never moist or wet.

Seeds are a rare find in the highest-quality cannabis, so if you find one be sure to set it aside for your own garden, assuming you are able to legally grow cannabis where you live.

Data should be available on the strains that you are interested in buying so that you can understand the various qualities of each product. Always look for test results from a trusted third-party laboratory.

Cannabis Pipe

There are myriad pipes to choose from at any cannabis dispensary, and whether you're beginning your journey or have a bit more experience, it's often wise to start with something small and relatively easy to use. You probably don't want to purchase equipment that's better suited for experienced users, like a big bong or other glassware. Also consider what type of material you would like your pipe to be made from, as there are options such as glass, plastic, metal, and even

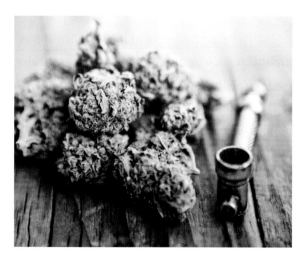

wood that can vary in storage capacity and ease of cleaning.

A small handheld pipe is a great start for beginners. These pipes typically fit in the palm of your hand and are ideal for casual, intermittent smoking when you're just beginning. Good-quality hand pipes are generally inexpensive and can range from a very plain-looking piece to an absolutely gorgeous blown-glass piece that will be the envy of your friends. Some smaller glass hand pipes can be exceptionally difficult to clean and you may have to consider rinsing yours with nail polish remover or acetone (and then thoroughly rinsing again to remove any toxic residues) if you want to keep it looking new and beautiful inside and out. Some people regularly run their pipes through the dishwasher while others allow the resin to accumulate inside the pipe because it contains concentrated cannabinoids that they find enjoyable.

Keep in mind that glass pipes can break easily. It's important to be particularly careful with someone else's glassware, because it's terrible etiquette to break a beloved pipe. Even though a small pipe holds a particular unassuming allure, consider using a pipe that has enough distance between the bowl and the mouthpiece to make it easy to light and also to keep the smoke cool as it travels toward your mouth. Cooler smoke results in less irritation to the airways, too—another boon.

If a vintage look appeals to you, you might also consider purchasing an old-fashioned gentleman's pipe; it will work just as well as any other hand pipe meant for smoking bud. Old-fashioned wooden pipes can also contribute a distinct flavor that other pipes may not have, and they can be a fun way to switch up your routine.

Water Pipe

Some experienced cannabis users will upgrade from using an old hand pipe to a water pipe, also known as a bong. Water pipes have a percolation chamber, which converts the smoke into water

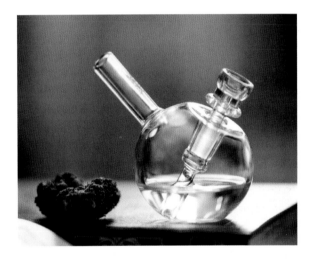

vapor, a process that can lessen the heat and harshness of the smoke so that there is less respiratory irritation. Water pipes come in all different shapes and sizes, making it a lot of fun to select one. Prices can range from a few dollars to several thousand, depending on the quality of the product and the customization of the glasswork.

You can easily find an inexpensive water pipe to suit your needs without a lot of fuss and extra details. Even though water pipes are available in plastic and metal, glassware is still the preferred medium for most experienced smokers.

One-Hitter

For the on-the-go smoker who doesn't want to use a vaporizer, one-hitters are also available. These are typically created from metal and are packed with flowers and smoked like a cigarette. They are useful when you want to be discreet in your cannabis consumption.

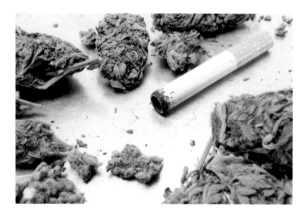

Rolling Paper

These days, almost all rolling papers are derived from Perpignan in the south of France. The small, light, thin leaves of paper have become popular and are made from materials like hemp rice, straw flax, or wood pulp. They range in size, length, and thickness as well as in the type of glue used to seal the paper. All these variations will have an effect on how your cannabis cigarette burns.

You can buy papers that have been bleached or left unbleached, based on your personal preference. Sometimes chemicals—such as calcium carbonate, chlorine, or potassium nitrate—are added to the papers to make them lighter, stronger, and more resistant to burning. However, those chemicals can make their way into your inhalations and cause irritation and even damage to the upper airways.

When choosing a rolling paper for yourself, it's important to be aware of both the size and flavor of the paper, as well as the ease of use. Rolling papers come in several sizes. In general, larger rolling papers are recommended, if you're going to be sharing your cannabis cigarette with two or more people. For ease and convenience, you may be tempted to roll a larger cigarette just for yourself to smoke on more than one occasion. However, to get the best flavor, many experienced cannabis users prefer to smoke fresh green cannabis, rather than cannabis that is partly ashy. So you may opt to have some smaller papers on hand for private consumption, as well as some larger papers for shared experiences.

It's wise to avoid flavored rolling papers, because even though many flavorings have been tested and proven to be safe for oral ingestion and breakdown through the GI tract, they have not been tested for safety when inhaled.

Another consideration is the cut of the paper. Some rolling papers are specifically designed to make the process of rolling simple and easy, even if you have very little experience or limited function in your hands and fingers due to arthritis.

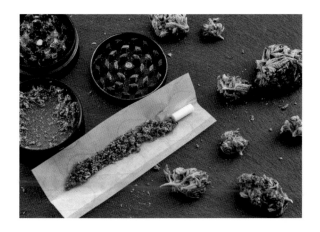

Rolling a cannabis cigarette is less of a science and more of an art. Many users enjoy that part of the process as much as consuming the product itself. There are a number of different well-known and several lesser-known brands of rolling papers to try. Whatever size or flavor of paper you choose will help you to curate a unique consumption experience for yourself.

Tincture or Edible

Unless you are an experienced cannabis aficionado, you should take your time with these products. Onset of action is often unreliable with tinctures and edibles; the peak of action can occur 60 to 90 minutes after administration. Many times the extent and intensity of the effect is unpredictable and difficult to control. Because of the delayed onset of action, some people assume that they haven't taken enough and then, with additional administration, often find they have taken too much. Virtually every one of my experienced cannabis patients has a negative story to share about an experience with an edible. So start slowly. It may take several attempts to determine what dosage is right for you.

NOTE: Please be very cautious about administering an edible and make sure that you are in a safe environment with someone you trust. Be sure to store edibles in a cool place and out of the reach of anyone under the age of 21.

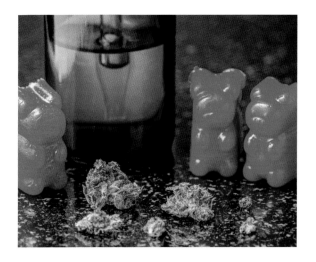

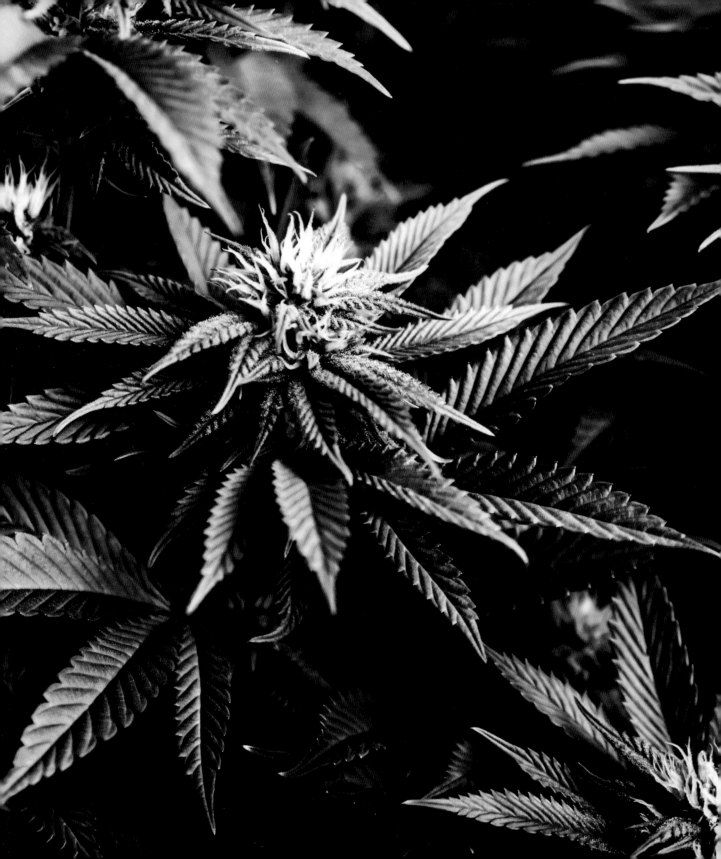

PART 5

< **Power Healers** >

CANNABIS STRAINS AND THEIR HEALTH BENEFITS

Whether you are using cannabis for relaxation after a long, stressful day, for general well-being, or as a focused treatment for anxiety or pain, there are numerous cannabis strains to choose from. Before settling on one or more strains, discuss your needs and how you intend to use the products with a cannabis-savvy professional. The strains listed in the following pages are ones I have used and that have been beneficial both to my patients and to myself.

Because the effects of each strain are different for every individual, I never recommend a specific strain for any condition. I always determine the strain and dosage based on a person's unique medical history and symptoms.

ACDC

ACDC isn't just one of my favorite hard-rock bands from the '80s; it's also one of my favorite Sativa-dominant strains in the medical cannabis toolkit. It provides a clearheaded, limited amount of intoxication while still providing deep relaxation to both mind and muscles. People find that it's effective for all kinds of medical conditions, especially if a high level of muscle relaxation or a deep level of mental relaxation without a lot of intoxication would be helpful. So if you're looking for a product that's going to leave you relatively clearheaded but with a lot of muscle relaxation, ACDC might be a great product for you.

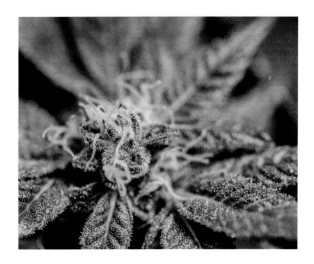

< 33 >

Chemdawg

Even though many of the products I recommend are suitable for anyone who's just starting out, some products should be used only by people who have very significant underlying conditions or who have used cannabinoid formulations for a long time. One of those products is Chemdawg, a Sativa hybrid with an unknown lineage, although its roots may be similar to those of OG Kush and Sour Diesel strains. Chemdawg is a high-THC, super-stinky, very potent product that creates a heavy body buzz and a heavily mind-altering, cerebral experience. It's a lasting one, too, so you don't need much, and it's definitely not for beginners.

Chernobyl

If you're seeking something with a rapid onset of action but a short duration, Chernobyl is a nice strain. It's a Sativa-dominant product that can have an average or even high amount of THC. Chernobyl has a great, creamy-sweet flavor, like a vanilla cookie, vanilla lemon ice, or lime sherbet. People love the taste of Chernobyl. The strain delivers a deep, relaxing body buzz along with a very potent head high. You may need to take it frequently if you're using it for treatment.

Cherry Pie

(See Harlequin, page 36.)

Crimea Blue

If you're seeking a strain that has real potential, look closely at Crimea Blue. In general, people who have used this strain describe the experience as happy—even euphoric—and relaxing. A few patients who have very significant nerve or muscle disease, have reported significant reduction in their symptoms with the use of Crimea Blue. I think we'll see more of it in the future.

Crystal Coma

As an internal-medicine doctor, I prefer to avoid using medications that are described as "crippling" or "debilitating," in terms of the level of relaxation they offer, but in some cases, when people are dealing with extreme physical pain or disability, the only way to really feel good is to dissociate entirely from the difficulties they are experiencing.

That's where Crystal Coma comes into play. It's a Sativa-dominant, 26-percent-THC hybrid that works very well to create a deep, trancelike experience that gives users profound relief from their conditions, at least for a short period. This strain is very potent and should probably be used only at the end of the day.

Death Star

Death Star is a strain that really lives up to its name. It builds in intensity over time and creates a very nice, euphoric experience, offering both a deep body buzz and a cerebral buzz. However, the strain has a fuel-y, skunky odor, an indication that you'll be left with at least some clarity of thinking after you've used the product, so that you can continue to function while controlling a condition.

Dr. Grinspoon

I'm sure most doctors—and most people, for that matter—would love to be remembered for having made a significant contribution to the well-being of others. If you're a doctor, for example, your legacy might be based on a particular surgical procedure that you developed and that was named after you. That actually happened to Dr. Lester Grinspoon, a professor at Harvard Medical School and also a medical cannabis advocate for 40 years. His product, a Sativa heirloom, was originally produced in Amsterdam and is highly coveted and prized for its long-lasting, cerebral high that leads to a lot of introspective thinking. I'm sure that Dr. Grinspoon approves.

Durban Poison

I always enjoy my conversations with patients who have been using medical cannabis formulations for a long time. They often know the industry as well, if not better, than I do. Durban Poison is one strain that these patients consistently recommend. Durban Poison comes from South Africa. It's a pure Sativa, and it's described as an energizing, euphoric, creative head high with virtually no body buzz or fatigue. This strain

is desirable when you're dealing with a variety of chronic conditions or if you are just in the mood to experience a sky-high head high. The adjectives used to describe the flavor of this popular strain include *sweet*, *licoricelike*, and even *minty*.

Euphoria

If you're looking for a medicinal cultivar that will leave you feeling socially engaged, uplifted, and excited, consider Euphoria. It's a Sativa strain that's not very well known and is somewhat difficult to find, but it does provide a high level of energy. As a side note, this strain is particularly easy to grow at home.

G-13

This strain is not only interesting because of the way that it makes you feel—there's also an intriguing backstory about how it was developed and why it is still accessible today. G-13 is

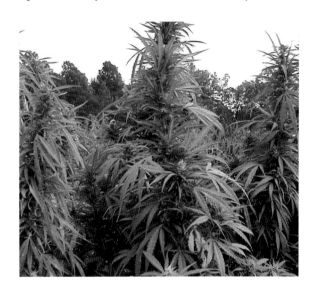

one of the original strains of cannabis, grown at the University of Mississippi, which happens to be the only facility in the United States where research can be done on cannabis—but only on one cultivar.

The story is that someone who was working at the University of Mississippi carried off just a single cutting of G-13 and was able to grow the plant and replicate the strain from that cutting. G-13 is supposed to provide a wonderful, uplifting, clear-headed high with a nice, deep body buzz and very limited fatigue. People also report that they love how it tastes—spicy and sweet.

Ghost

Ghost, a combination of Indica and Sativa, is a middle-of-the-road hybrid of uncertain lineage, although, judging from its appearance, it's likely a close relative of OG Kush. It creates a cheerful, uplifting high and has a wonderful piney, citrusy flavor. It's suitable for times when you want to be relaxed but still social—calm and controlled but not to the point of wanting to withdraw and rest.

Girl Scout Cookie

For a great, everyday high that's tolerated well by amateurs and regular cannabis consumers alike, Girl Scout Cookie is an excellent option. The product is Sativa-dominant and has an amazing lineage, with both OG Kush and the famed and coveted Durban Poison in its background. Aptly named Girl Scout Cookie, the product is well liked by everybody for

its fruity, sweet, and sometimes mildly spicy flavor. Use it for an uplifting, sociable high that will also give you a great, deep sleep two or three hours after your inhalations, thanks to the generous amount of the cannabinoid CBN in the strain.

Godfather OG

Godfather OG is a very strong and valuable medical cannabis cultivar. It's a potent Indica hybrid with THC percentages that range up to 28 percent. Godfather OG is a cross between Grapes and OG Kush, so the flavoring is very pleasant. It creates a potent head high with full body relaxation and a serious case of the munchies.

Grapes

For a strong Indica hybrid with a high CBD content, Grapes is an excellent choice to help stabilize mood as well as alleviate many medical conditions, including anxiety and stress. It delivers a strong, tranquil experience that is relatively fog-free and has a great green-grape, grape soda, or bubblegum flavor.

Harlequin

I recommend Harlequin to my patients who use medical cannabis all the time. I use it interchangeably with Cherry Pie, because of the similar THC and CBD ratios. Both strains are high in CBD and fairly low in THC, so people who use them can get a considerable amount of relaxation and relief from symptoms without a lot of

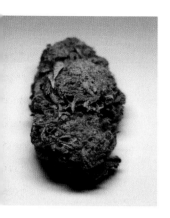

intoxication. The nice thing about both strains is that each has a different terpene profile, so your response will be a little different, depending on which strain you use. Cherry Pie is the sweeter of the two and a little bit citrusy, while Harlequin has a somewhat earthier, musky aroma. These high-CBD, low-THC products are very good for many chronic medical conditions, and they are also a boon for general relaxation and mood stabilization when you'd like to avoid a significant psychoactive effect.

Haze

Developed in Monterey, California, in the 1970s, Haze is another very potent Sativa hybrid that gives an all-consuming cerebral high. The strain is sometimes referred to as "ampheta-weed" because of its psychedelic effects. Be sure to use it only with a high level of caution and a considerable amount of experience under your belt. This is not a product for beginners.

Headband

A number of my patients tell me they experience a stiffening sensation in their neck or shoulders when they use some cannabinoid formulations. Apparently Headband creates a sensation of tightness around the head and neck, especially in the jaw and around the ears. Everybody has a slightly different reaction to this strain, but the overall effect is delightful; it's an interesting physical phenomenon worth experiencing. Headband is a combination of OG Kush and Sour Diesel, so it has a very nice lineage and a wonderful floral, piney flavor, with just a hint of diesel, as you might expect. The strain delivers a happy, uplifted, cerebral buzz, followed quickly by a full-body high. It's a classic creeper weed that's going to sneak up on you, though, so be aware of that as you consume this product.

Jack Herer

Known as the champagne of hemp, Jack Herer is an excellent strain for both novices and experienced consumers of cannabis. It's a Sativa-dominant hybrid named after Jack Herer—he was sometimes called the emperor of hemp and is considered the father of modern cannabis advocacy. Herer is also the author of *The Emperor Wears No Clothes*, a book that is often cited in efforts to decriminalize and legalize cannabis. The product has a lemony, zesty, sweet flavor, and, as mentioned, it is well tolerated by consumers of all levels. It creates a clear, long-lasting, creativity-promoting head high. It was designed in the Netherlands in the 1990s.

Kosher Kush

Kosher Kush is another of my favorites among medicinal herbs. It's aptly named because it was initially developed by a group of Jewish growers and referred to as "Jews' Gold," but Kosher Kush is the name that stuck. It's a mild Indica hybrid that creates a relaxed, spacey body buzz along with a very calming cerebral buzz that leads to eventual deep sleep and a serious case of the munchies shortly after consumption.

Lavender

Lavender is almost as sweet as the flower itself. It's an Indica-dominant hybrid and has a wonderful violet hue. Many people who have used Lavender report that it's the best mellow, cerebral buzz experience around and also generates a very nice, relaxing body buzz.

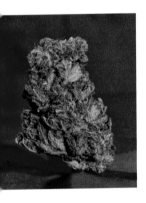

Mazar

Mazar (rhymes with *bizarre*) is a powerfully sedative strain with an immobilizing narcotic effect and should be used only if you've had experience with other strains of cannabinoids that offer a similar mind-warping experience.

Medicine Man

Medicine Man, also known as White Rhino, is an extremely popular medicinal strain that has a history, anecdotally, of offering relief for virtually every condition typically treated with cannabis formulations, including stress, anxiety, pain, and insomnia. Medicine Man is a high-Indica hybrid, so it's best not to use it if you're planning to be particularly productive. Use it, instead, during leisure periods. The formulation is high in THC and also high in CBD, so you can expect a lot of relaxation but also a lot of creative thinking.

NYC Diesel

NYC Diesel, a kind of Sour Diesel, is a favorite among New York City dwellers who are looking to be productive, cheerful, creative, motivated, and socially engaged with other people throughout their day. This formulation has a great fruity, lemony aroma and works very well to create a pleasurable, uplifting high along with a relaxing body buzz that allows the user to enjoy an extremely busy workday. It is massively popular for use in daytime, precisely because it doesn't hamper productivity—and may actually improve it. So if you're looking for a fun daytime recreational strain to use while getting a lot of serious work done, this one may be perfect.

OG Kush

OG Kush is an Indica-dominant hybrid that deserves special mention for so many reasons. It has a surprisingly high level of CBN (cannabinol), which produces a gentle, sedative high, a wonderful trancelike state that helps the user drift off to sleep several hours after inhaling the product. OG Kush has been the backbone of the cannabis industry on the West Coast and has contributed to the development of so many other great cultivars and formulations. In fact, OG Kush prerolls are available for purchase in virtually every consumption lounge. It's one of the few strains that's consistently available in a pre-roll so that it's ready and easy to use for anyone who wants to enjoy the experience. It stimulates a really nice appetite after a few hours, too.

Purple Kush

I love to recommend Purple Kush, an almost pure Indica, not only for the deep body buzz and the very intense, blissful, euphoric, and cerebral relaxation it offers, but for its significant medical benefits as well. For example, in the end stages of a neurological disease like ALS (Lou Gehrig's disease) or MS (multiple sclerosis), swallowing can become very difficult and can result in recurrent lung infections. Drying the mouth with Purple Kush can provide real relief in those situations.

Red Congo

Everybody's looking for a little more optimism and motivation nowadays. Right? Red Congo, also known as Red Congolese, is a spirit-lifting and mind-sharpening Sativa that provides exactly those. People who use this popular strain describe a smoke that tastes sweet and pungent with citrus notes; it also promotes focus and a bright outlook. You can get a lot of work done while on this product, so consider it primarily for daytime use.

Romulan

This pine- and pepper-scented strain is the stuff of legend in Canada. The strain has an interesting lineage, too, with roots that go back to Africa, Korea, and Colombia. It creates a deeply intense cerebral buzz with one of the most intense couch-locking body buzzes in the industry. Enjoy Romulan when you're ready to stay at home!

Skunk

Skunk's captivating, mysterious global lineage, along with its development in the psychedelic 1970s and its contribution to so many other great strains, have made it one of the best medicinal products available. And for so many reasons. It works incredibly well to generate a cheerful, relaxed euphoria and a nice, deep, relaxing body buzz. In addition to that, the strain creates an intense experience of the munchies for people who have difficulty stimulating their appetite.

Skunk by itself is amazing, but you can look for all kinds of other products that have this particular cannabis strain in their lineage, such as Ultra Skunk, Skunk Passion, and Orange Bud, for a slightly different experience that still give you all the benefits of Skunk.

Sour Diesel

(See NYC Diesel, page 38.)

Sunset Sherbet

With its powerful, relaxing body buzz and jolt of cerebral clarity and energy, Sunset Sherbet is one of Dr. Mary's favorites because it is so valuable in social settings for creating a relaxed, cheerful, talkative—even euphoric—atmosphere. Socializing—having time to relax and enjoy the company of friends—is not only very important for your personal happiness; it also improves the quality of your life, which can certainly help extend it. Sunset Sherbet, among other recreational favorites, such as NYC Diesel and OG Kush, does a good job of making important social experiences extremely relaxing and enjoyable. The high-THC as well as the high-CBD content in this strain—a cross between Girl Scout Cookie and Blackberry Kush—confers a great many benefits, thanks to its powerful lineage.

Tangie

Developed in the 1990s in Amsterdam, Tangie is a Sativa hybrid that you'll best enjoy before spending an evening with friends. It creates an uplifting, relaxing buzz suitable for socializing.

Trainwreck

A Sativa-dominant hybrid developed in Humboldt County, California, in the 1980s, Trainwreck hits hard and fast, just as its name suggests. The strain has a peppery citrus flavor, with a little bit of fuel or diesel in the background. A mutt, Trainwreck's lineage can be traced to Afghani products and a mix of Thai and Mexican strains that create a significant amount of focus—almost a hyperfocus. For people who have difficulty concentrating and can't seem to get their thoughts organized, Trainwreck can be surprisingly helpful.

Wedding Cake

Wedding Cake is a popular and easy-to-find Indica hybrid. Although the THC content in this strain is extremely high, it doesn't create a seriously psychedelic experience in the least. Instead it delivers a really lovely body buzz and a cheerful, euphoric head high, and it tastes fantastic. Wedding Cake is appropriately named because it tastes like sweet berries with a little bit of vanilla flavor, which makes it a very easy product to consume. It also has an extremely long-lasting effect.

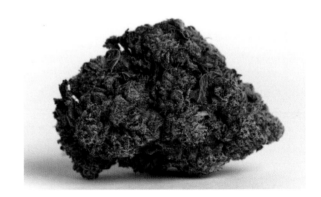

ABOUT DOSING—An Important Note from the Authors

In this book you'll note that we refrain from giving recommendations for dosing. The reasons are few but vital. While dosage of CBD, which heals without a high, can be self-modulated, or titrated, without debilitating side effects, dosage of THC is different. Hippies from the 1960s and '70s, and even yuppies from the '80s, used cannabis with relatively low levels of THC. "Good shit"—now the name of a brand of seed—was a general term for a cannabis that delivered a mellow high and could be enjoyed frequently with little other harm, other than getting the munchies and "being out of it" for a while. Today, however, sophisticated breeding can produce plants with THC so high that users experience dependency and even toxic reactions. Always confer with a cannabis-savvy physician about products and dosing before adding cannabis to your medical regimen, whether for treating a serious condition, such as Crohn's disease, or for general well-being.

You are about to begin an extraordinary journey that originated in a time so ancient that we cannot put a date to it and progressed to an era so scientifically cutting-edge that we only have to dream our vision of cannabis as a healer to make it happen. Join the journey with optimism, creative thinking, scientific caution, and, above all, ultimate respect for this sacred plant and your sacred body.

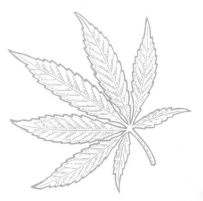

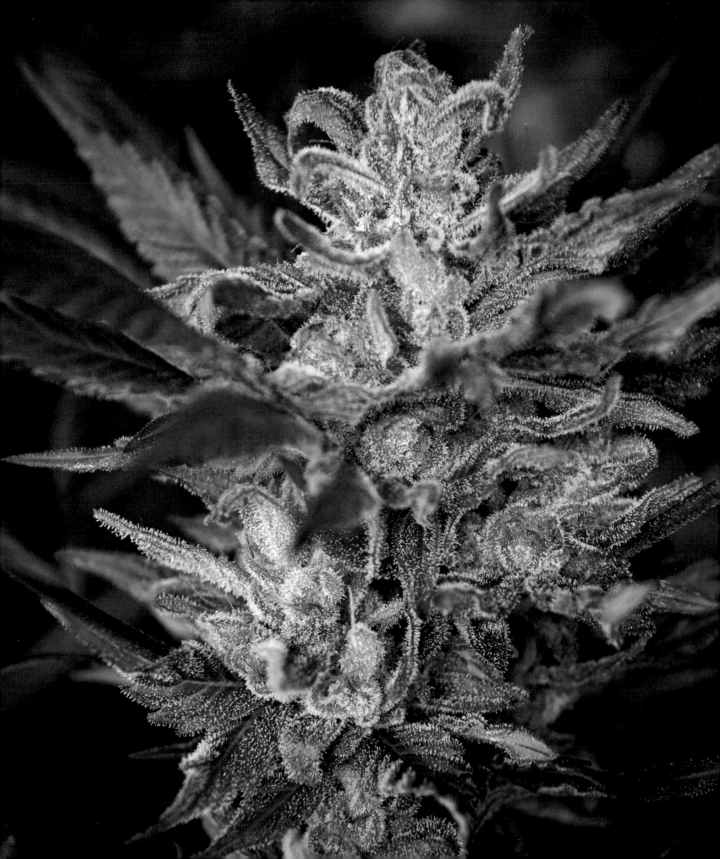

PART 6

< Power Healing with Cannabis >

TREATMENTS FOR 33 CONDITIONS

Now that you've discovered the basics about cannabis and its health benefits, this section will give you insights into specific conditions and how cannabis may be in your future as a healer and messenger of long-lasting health and wellness.

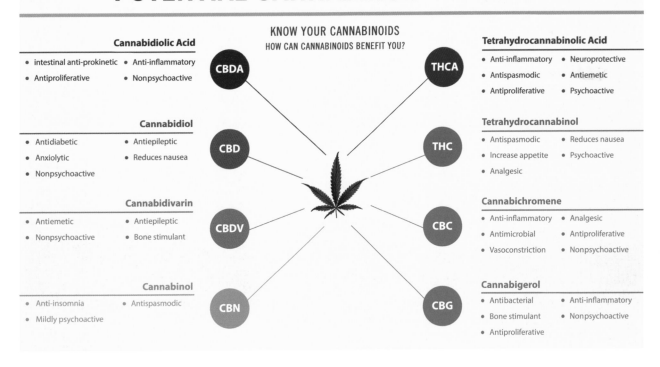

POTENTIAL CANNABINOID BENEFITS

KNOW YOUR CANNABINOIDS
HOW CAN CANNABINOIDS BENEFIT YOU?

Cannabidiolic Acid — CBDA
- intestinal anti-prokinetic
- Antiproliferative
- Anti-inflammatory
- Nonpsychoactive

Cannabidiol — CBD
- Antidiabetic
- Anxiolytic
- Nonpsychoactive
- Antiepileptic
- Reduces nausea

Cannabidivarin — CBDV
- Antiemetic
- Nonpsychoactive
- Antiepileptic
- Bone stimulant

Cannabinol — CBN
- Anti-insomnia
- Mildly psychoactive
- Antispasmodic

Tetrahydrocannabinolic Acid — THCA
- Anti-inflammatory
- Antispasmodic
- Antiproliferative
- Neuroprotective
- Antiemetic
- Psychoactive

Tetrahydrocannabinol — THC
- Antispasmodic
- Increase appetite
- Analgesic
- Reduces nausea
- Psychoactive

Cannabichromene — CBC
- Anti-inflammatory
- Antimicrobial
- Vasoconstriction
- Analgesic
- Antiproliferative
- Nonpsychoactive

Cannabigerol — CBG
- Antibacterial
- Bone stimulant
- Antiproliferative
- Anti-inflammatory
- Nonpsychoactive

< 43 >

1) Accidents

An accident can be as simple as stubbing your toe or slicing into a finger when you're cutting potatoes. Even a simple accident is unexpected—and, to an extent, alarming. More tragic events—such as serious car accidents and drug overdoses—can leave lifelong scars, both physical and psychological, and, worse yet, bring on death. The most common causes of death from accidents are by poisoning and drug overdose, with some 64,695 such deaths reported in the United States in 2017. Motor vehicle accidents are the next most common cause of death: 34,247 fatal events took place in the United States in 2017, with 37,133 related deaths. Falls come in third, with 36,338 deaths. Causes of other fatal accidents include inhalation—such as drowning and smoke inhalation—and exposure to extreme heat or extreme cold.

Motor vehicle accidents can usually be prevented if you follow safe driving guidelines. Number one: Stay sober. Every country around the world has a zero-tolerance policy on driving while intoxicated. Sobriety is assessed by two measures: response time and lane weave. *Response time* is the time it takes for you to hit the brake so you can safely swerve around another car or avoid hitting something in front of you. *Lane weave* is the frequency of weaving between lanes. While sober, drivers should be traveling in a relatively straight line between the middle and outside lane markings. Intoxicated drivers often weave between them. Prolonged response time and lane weave are two main indicators that a driver is impaired—and they're important pieces of evidence in a sobriety test.

In the case of drugs, poisoning and overdose accidents continue to cause serious problems in virtually every community across the United States. Nearly one-third of opioid deaths in New York state involve prescription opioids.

Current Treatments

Avoiding an accident in the first place should be a priority. That means never consuming alcohol or intoxicating medications when you plan to drive, operate machinery, or even walk across the street. For anyone with an alcohol or drug addiction, medications and other support are available. (See "Addiction and Withdrawal," page 46.) For those with muscle weakness and spasms or attention deficit challenges, reaction to a potential emergency can be uncontrolled or too slow. Again, in those instances, medications and other support can help. (See "Multiple Sclerosis," page 117; "Parkinson's Disease," page 125; and "ADHD," page 49.)

Why CBD or Medical Cannabis Might Be the Answer

Cannabis and cannabinoid formulations can reduce the risk of accidents. A study on synthetic cannabinoid formulations and their effect on driving, published in 2018 in the journal *Brain and Behavior*, showed no increase in risk of motor vehicle accidents with the use of cannabis formulations in people with multiple sclerosis or other serious muscular disorders. Pharmaceutical companies worldwide have accumulated 55,000 patient years of information (based on an established calculation) on driving safety while using synthetic cannabinoids, and no driving impairment or safety risk has emerged—not even an increased risk of parking tickets! It looks as though people who use cannabinoid formulations drive safely and park safely.

Studies also show that cannabis can help curtail drug accidents. In 2016, the *Clinical Journal of Pain* published the results of a six-month-long Israeli clinical study of 206 patients previously treated with opioid formulations; they were subsequently treated, in the study, with cannabinoid formulations—either in the form of cigarettes or cookies—three times a day. The patients' opioid use decreased by 44 percent. Just three months later, after follow-up appointments, doctors reported that of the 73 patients who had been on opioids at baseline (that is, at the beginning of the study), 32 were able to completely discontinue their opioid treatment.

SUPPORTING RESEARCH

In the case of driving, a person's response time and lane weave are increased when alcohol and cannabis are used in combination. An increase in response time can also happen when a person is taking sedating medications, such as antidepressants and benzodiazepines, which are usually prescribed for insomnia, anxiety, or depression. However, researchers have found that after just two weeks, a driver on a sedating antidepressant showed little difference in driving capabilities from a driver on a placebo. There appears to be a similar tolerance when drivers use cannabinoid formulations on a regular basis, meaning that cannabis alone may not have a significant impact on driving. In fact, the only evidence we have seen that cannabinoid formulations cause problems during driving is when they are combined with alcohol. That's when you can really see changes in response time and lane weave.

In addition, when you treat certain conditions, such as ADHD, with stimulants like Adderall® —which help a person focus—driving skills will improve. The same has been shown to be true in treating multiple sclerosis patients with spasm-controlling medications, including cannabinoid formulations. Again, it is important to remember that the United States, and every other country around the world, has a zero-tolerance policy for driving while intoxicated. Always avoid driving under the influence of cannabis or cannabinoid formulations or any other products that could limit your ability to be a safe and effective driver.

Amazingly, the decrease in alcohol consumption in states where cannabis is legal for recreational use has resulted in a decrease in traffic accidents! In studies examining the relationship between traffic fatalities, alcohol consumption, and the passage of legislation legalizing recreational cannabis in different states, researchers have found that recreational cannabis legalization is associated with a decrease in sales of beer; in reduced total alcohol consumption, particularly among adults; and in alcohol-related traffic fatalities. We have the potential to make a significant impact on the safety of our roads by legalizing cannabis nationwide.

In the case of drug-related accidents, data show that cannabinoid formulations can reduce the reliance on opioids—and reduce opioid overdose—for patients with chronic pain. Cannabis can also help ease chronic pain directly, thus reducing a patient's need for opioids in the first place. Not only does using medical cannabis benefit the person in pain, it diverts important opioid medication from people who misuse it for recreational purposes to people who really need it. The opioid epidemic could be a completely avoidable issue—especially if the availability of medical cannabis was widespread.

> *"I started using cannabis to try to reach the state of mind I had reached before with more dangerous drugs. At the time I started using, I was on methadone. Then I was able to ease off the methadone. Now cannabis is the only thing that makes me feel better. Using it, I can reach a zen-like state, and I don't need other drugs. I can find the state of mind I need with cannabis."*
>
> —Tony, 48, **Automotive Design Implementer**

Integrative Tip > > > > >

Avoiding accidents requires that you manage not only the external environment but your internal environment as well. To prevent falling as you age, remove loose rugs, so you don't trip, and make sure to exercise every day to strengthen your core, glutes, and quads. Keep sedating medications to a minimum and choose medicinals that will provide support for pain and sleep disorders without risk of overdose or excess sedation. Take medications as prescribed, and, just as important, choose nutritious foods for every meal.

2) Addiction and Withdrawal

America is a nation running on addiction—to alcohol, food, cigarettes, and now opioids—with little sign of letting up. But there is light on the horizon. Addiction has reached such epidemic proportions that physicians and scientists are making treatment a priority. Just look at the numbers: The CDC (Centers for Disease Control and Prevention) reports that alcohol abuse causes some 88,000 deaths a year, and in 2018, the CDC named smoking as the leading cause of preventable death for some 34.2 million Americans. Now opioids—including fentanyl, morphine, and oxycodone—are the up-and-coming competitors for those grim statistics: Since 2010 some 300,000 people have died from the use and abuse of opioids—and the medical care associated with that scourge has increased by 3,000 percent. In 2017, the CDC reported drug overdose as the leading cause of death in the United

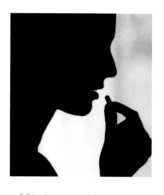

States—about 70,000 deaths per year—and made it a priority to escalate prevention and treatment efforts, stop trafficking, and generally raise public awareness. Still, drug addiction continues to contribute to death, disability, loss of productivity, and crime. People need to know—and care—about what's happening to their bodies. Basically, when any toxin is ingested, whether it is nicotine, opiates, alcohol, or processed foods, bodily systems—including the ECS (endocannabinoid system)—are under attack. This assault can lead to heart disease and lung cancer in smokers; cirrhosis of the liver and esophageal cancer in alcoholics; and overall system breakdown, including depression and suicide, in drug users. Interacting with ECS receptors, toxins can produce a happy high for a brief period and a feeling of reward. But those feelings dissipate within hours, and the desire for more drugs can resurface as an all-consuming craving.

Current Remedies

Methadone and Suboxone® are available to help people withdraw from opioids, but strict regulations govern the acquisition and use of those medications, which makes them somewhat hard to find. A new drug, naltrexone, has been approved by the FDA (Food and Drug Administration) for the NIH-approved treatment of alcohol and opioid addiction. Naltrexone can also ease disabling repetitive and self-injurious behaviors in some children and adults with autism.

Why CBD or Medical Cannabis Might Be the Answer

Preventing addiction in the first place is always preferable to treating it once it has you in its grip. CBD can help. When taken successfully to enhance sleep or lower inflammation, stress, insomnia, pain, anxiety, and the resulting depression, CBD guides the body toward an ongoing balance, making the immediate gratification derived from smoking, drinking alcohol, and taking drugs less sought after.

Opioid addiction usually begins when a person takes the drug to alleviate pain. The right amount connects with CB1 receptors as well as opioid receptors—which are found near one another in the ECS —to enhance well-being. Too much of the drug, however, is detrimental.

Studies conducted by researchers at Mount Sinai Hospital in New York City have shown that high doses of CBD can help lower cue-induced cravings that may occur when a user in withdrawal sees a friend using opioids or is in other situations linked to opioid use. Dr. Mary's patients have said that for the first couple of years after the drug is withdrawn, it is difficult to manage cue-induced cravings. For some, it can take up to two years to stop waking up in a cold sweat with intense cravings in the middle of the night. For others, such cravings can be overwhelming. In the Mount Sinai opioid study, researchers looked at 400mg of CBD, 800mg of CBD, and a placebo to test the most efficient means of reducing cue-induced cravings among patients. In all, 64.3 percent of the participants in the study had stopped using opioids only in the previous month and were experiencing anxiety associated with cue-induced cravings. (See "Anxiety," page 53.) CBD in either amount reduced their anxiety for a full week, with no increase in mortality or risk of intoxication.

In a 2014 study published in the *American Journal of Drug and Alcohol Abuse*, patients reported using cannabis in excess to experience altered perception, a sense of celebration, enjoyment of the drug with alcohol, and to help cope with boredom. Whatever the reason for use of cannabis, a 2015 report in the journal *Substance Abuse* noted several studies suggesting that CBD has "beneficial impact on the intoxication, addiction, and relapse phases of not only cannabis addiction but of tobacco and alcohol addiction as well."

SUPPORTING RESEARCH

One theory about how CBD may work to overcome addiction, ease symptoms of withdrawal, and avoid relapse centers on the big role that endocannabinoid receptors play in how we respond to rewards. The immediate reward a person feels upon taking a pill or a drink or having a smoke helps lead them down an addictive path. Studies increasingly show that CBD may play a role in blocking the receptors that produce that feeling of reward. It is also likely that CBD helps stop the uptake of serotonin, allowing it to remain in the body long enough to help relieve the anxiety and insomnia that accompany withdrawal. While the endocannabinoid system is central to the addicting sensation of reward, it is fortunate that it also helps reset brain circuitry and promote healing. CBD is a key player in both of those pathways.

" *When I look back, I was taking 15 to 20 pills a day. My medicine cabinet was full of bottles. I was consistently 3 to 4 out of 10, in pain, on high-dose opiates, and now it's 5 out of 10 with cannabis, which is very tolerable, given what I've been through with illnesses and injury. It's manageable. I took opiates for 13 years, initially ibuprofen, then tramadol, then OxyContin®, and morphine tablets. I felt like I was there, but I was just a shell of myself. I got a new primary care doctor and she recommended that I get a medical cannabis card. I got pretty high at first, but I worked on strain selection and after 30 days I began to feel alive again.* **"**

—Jennifer, 45, Cosmetologist

Hyla Cass, MD

After graduating from the University of Toronto School of Medicine, Dr. Hyla Cass interned at Los Angeles County–USC Medical Center and completed a psychiatric residency at Cedars-Sinai Medical Center/UCLA. Today Dr. Cass is based in Los Angeles and has a virtual consulting practice. A nationally acclaimed innovator and expert in the fields of integrative medicine, psychiatry, and addiction recovery, Dr. Cass helps individuals to take charge of their health, withdraw from psychiatric medication, and overcome substance abuse with the aid of natural supplements, including her own brand of hemp oil extract. Dr. Cass follows these principles "to help heal our health care system, our planet, and ultimately ourselves":

- Treat the whole person—mind, body, spirit, and environment.
- Determine the deepest root causes of symptoms, using scientific lab testing, if needed.
- Apply a continuum of treatments, always beginning with the safest and most natural possible.

Integrative Tip >>>>>

A 2020 edition of the journal *Psychological Science* cautions patients to avoid stressful situations when fighting addiction. In a supporting study from New South Wales, Australia, researchers reported that patients under cognitive stress or fatigue were more easily tempted by unwanted environmental cues. Social and emotional support are also key to resisting the temptation to use drugs when under stress. A 2012 study across 142 nations concluded that support—especially from a dependable friend or family member—reduced an addict's negative feelings and improved general well-being, lowering the need for other joy-inducing factors.

3) ADHD

Attention-deficit/hyperactivity disorder, or ADHD, can haunt an individual for life, compromising early learning as well as long-term social interactions and well-being. However, early detection and treatment can have beneficial long-term effects. The American Psychiatric Association (APA) has identified three types of ADHD that affect children's behavior in different ways. Predominantly inattentive ADHD impacts girls more than boys and involves daydreaming and challenges with focusing, finishing tasks, and following instructions. Children whose ADHD is predominantly characterized as hyperactive-impulsive are attentive but fidgety, are prone to interrupt, and act impulsively. The third type of ADHD is characterized by a combination of impulsive and hyperactive behaviors as well as inattention. What brings on ADHD? Researchers aren't sure, but it may begin in the brain, perhaps with lower levels of dopamine, a soothing chemical that also plays a part in movement and emotional responses. On the other hand, the onset of ADHD may be due to a brain structure in which the areas wired for movement and self-control are smaller than usual. Some have theorized that genetics, premature birth, and environmental toxins may play a role. While ADHD is often diagnosed in school-age children—twice as often in boys as in girls—individuals may also be diagnosed with ADHD as adults. The bad-good news is that while about 60 percent of children will still have symptoms as adults, their symptoms often dissipate with age. With treatment, life can be enjoyable and focused, but without it, an adult may be challenged by a lifetime of forgetfulness, poor time management, and impatience that negatively impacts work and personal life. Treating ADHD with medication, behavioral therapy, or both depends on age of diagnosis and will change as a person grows older. You may wonder: What about ADD? Attention deficit disorder is simply the outdated term for the milder, predominantly inattentive form of ADHD.

Current Remedies

There are three categories of pharmaceuticals that address ADHD: stimulants, such as dextroamphetamine (Adderall) and methylphenidate (Ritalin®), which help with focus and are used to treat about 80 percent of patients; milder nonstimulants that promote concentration and impulse control; and antidepressants, which help to address symptoms of anxiety and depression. All three of these categories of pharmaceuticals may also have side effects, including insomnia, stomachache, mood swings, and psychiatric conditions.

Why CBD or Medical Cannabis Might Be the Answer

We don't have randomized controlled trials on children with ADHD using cannabis to control their condition, but a very smart study by a group of Duke University researchers, published by the Public Library of Science in a 2016 *PLOS ONE* journal, is interesting. The researchers studied 268 chat rooms across a wide range of platforms on the internet in order to find out what people were saying about taking cannabis for ADHD. The results? Most people said they were able to sit still for longer periods and could concentrate longer if they used cannabis to treat their symptoms. Those findings support the image you would actually see in a functional MRI or PET scan, showing how various areas of the brain respond to cannabis. A PET scan definitely shows that cannabis affects the areas in the back of the brain—the brain stem and the cerebellum—which control movement, much as methylphenidate or dextroamphetamine do.

Once someone can just sit still long enough to resolve hyperactivity, a lot of their attention deficit can be relieved, too.

A case study from Finland, published by *Karger* in 2018, followed a patient who was diagnosed at age 33 with ADHD. After five years, researchers concluded that a THC-rich medication helped alleviate the patient's frustration and angry outbursts and improved his ability to focus. A second mixture of THC and CBD not only helped subdue unwanted side effects from the THC medication but also improved sleep. Cannabis luminary and neurologist Dr. Ethan Russo has worked with children with ADHD for more than 15 years and has noted that "controlled trials of cannabis medicines for children and adults with ADHD seem clearly indicated."

SUPPORTING RESEARCH

The ECS (endocannabinoid system), with its CB1 and CB2 receptors and endocannabinoids anandamide and 2-AG, interacts with the central nervous system, a key player in ADHD. Dr. David Bearman, a pioneer in cannabis research and a longtime advocate of substance abuse programs, has led the way in studying how cannabinoids interact with the ECS to affect ADHD. His work suggests that cannabinoids—whether produced inside the body or supplemented from the outside—support the release of dopamine in the body. Dopamine, in turn, helps the brain regulate information input while promoting calm

and focus. His work, as well as Dr. Russo's, is supported in the 2018 case study in the journal *Medical Cannabis and Cannabinoids*.

"*I used to use Ritalin, but I found that it decreased my energy and creativity. I felt that it was squelching my vibrancy and liveliness. My life was dulled down. Cannabis has really helped manage my hyperactivity, and I've also tried to be more patient with myself.***"**

—Sondra, 42, Author

Integrative Tip >>>>>
Creating small, tangible goals for a child, then rewarding that behavior may help them gradually gain focus. Parent-teacher collaboration can be key. In one instance, a student was "graded" every 20 minutes for successfully sitting at his desk, focusing on an assignment, and respectfully interacting with fellow students. His reward: extra time playing basketball after school. There's more. Staying outside to play for at least 20 minutes has been shown to improve concentration. So, in this way, parents and teachers can work together by rewarding sedentary behavior in schools with plenty of outdoor exercise after school.

4) ALS

Amyotrophic lateral sclerosis (ALS) takes its name from the Greek term *amyotrophic*, meaning no ("a") muscle ("myo") nourishment ("trophic").

Without nourishment, a muscle atrophies, or wastes away. Also known as Lou Gehrig's disease, after the baseball legend who fought the disease on the world stage, ALS is a rare condition affecting just 5 to 7 in 100,000 adults. The cause of ALS? It appears to be inherited rarely, in about 10 percent of the population. But for the vast majority, there is no obvious environmental or genetic association. Cases simply occur sporadically, with no known history of the disease in the family. Scientists do know that the disease prompts the death of neurons, breaking through the protective myelin sheaths that surround them. This, in turn, prompts gradual muscle degeneration throughout the body, a process that eventually shuts down the movement of leg and arm muscles and limits the ability to swallow or breathe. Because of that loss of muscle control, a patient with ALS is forced to lie down or sit; consequently, muscle pain and spasticity focus in specific locations, causing intense pain. Appetite loss and depression also enter the picture. Swallowing becomes difficult, and extreme secretion of saliva is hard to manage, bringing more discomfort. Finally, bronchial tubes going from the throat to the lungs bring in less air. Gradually respiratory failure sets in. Today, the ALS Association and its partners are supporting exciting clinical trials that focus on gene and stem cell therapy. There is also a place for cannabis in the ongoing research into effective treatments.

Current Remedies

According to the ALS Association, recent scientific advancements in understanding the makeup, effects, and progression of the disease have led to the approval of four drugs, by the US FDA, to treat ALS: Rilutek®, Nuedexta®, Radicava®, and Tiglutik®. In addition to those drugs, other medications that address pain, depression, insomnia, and the accompanying symptoms are also available. As mentioned, the ALS Association is also funding global studies to develop new treatments that focus on gene and stem cell therapy. Scientists are reporting promising advancements. Studies reported by the American Academy of Neurology (AAN) show that participation in programs that include support groups and physical therapy at a multidisciplinary ALS clinic can help a patient manage their symptoms, improve their quality of life, and prolong their survival.

Why CBD or Medical Cannabis Might Be the Answer

ALS is one of the key conditions that can be well served by cannabis, wherever its use is legal for medical purposes. Many ALS symptoms, including muscle spasms and pain, respond well to medical cannabis, according to documentation. Data as far back as the 1980s show that cannabis also counters appetite loss and lifts mood.

In the case of ALS, the dry mouth that cannabis users experience actually helps patients who are having trouble managing oral secretions as the ability to swallow grows progressively weaker. Cannabis can also have a mild bronchodilator effect, opening the airways to the lungs as respiratory failure sets in, and can play a neuroprotective role by staving off neuron death and helping to maintain healthy myelin sheaths around degenerating neurons. All this can be a tremendous help to an ALS sufferer.

"When I don't have cannabis, I'm worse. When I do have it, I'm better. It stops my twitching, and it makes my throat stronger. It also helps with my depression. My throat needs to be strong because otherwise I choke, and I can't choke. There is not one medication that can do all of the things that this medication does."

—Alex, 54, Chemist

Integrative Tip >>>>>

Never underestimate the power of socializing. Being part of a support group, when facing any disease, is key to maintaining a good quality of life. In fact, experts hold that these groups are indispensable in treating the disease by giving both patients and caregivers opportunities to exchange information about key advancements in science and vital integrative therapies as well as share personal experiences. The camaraderie that grows from sharing feelings and emotions in a support group helps patients with ALS experience a better quality of life while living with the disease.

5) Anxiety

A bout of nerve-related nausea isn't uncommon among actors before walking onstage. It's a relatively normal stress response, and it dissipates as an actor's creative resilience takes over and the audience appears to fade behind the stage lights. But stressful events can also trigger long-standing nervous conditions in people who are vulnerable to them. Those conditions, known as mood disorders, can become disabling. Anxiety disorder, for example, is all too prevalent. According to the National Institute of Mental Health (NIMH), 18 percent of adults have symptoms of an anxiety disorder in any given year, but only a third of them receive treatment. In an increasingly stress-ridden world, children are also victims of anxiety. A 2018 study, reported in the journal *Medicines*, contends that anxiety disorders "represent the most prevalent mental illnesses in the world, with high societal costs." Anxiety disorders include generalized anxiety disorder, obsessive-compulsive disorder, panic disorder, social phobias, specific phobias, and post-traumatic stress disorder. These can be accompanied by any combination of shortness of

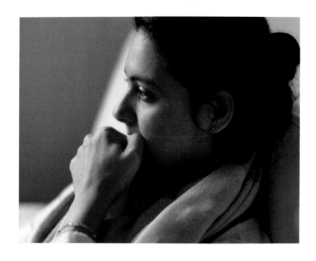

breath, chest pain, heart palpitations, sweating, and intense, paralyzing fear. Once triggered, these attacks can return again and again, becoming chronic and impossible to control. They may limit your ability to socialize, interact at work, or even shop for groceries in crowded aisles.

Another kind of anxiety is prompted by withdrawal from pharmaceuticals, especially antianxiety medications such as antidepressants, sedatives, and painkillers or opioids. Some patients have said that in the first couple of years after a drug is withdrawn, cue-induced triggers—such as seeing a drug-using friend or reliving a drug-related experience—can prompt a craving for that drug to the point of breaking out in a sweat and shaking. So strong is the addiction that many cannot fight it. The death of some 300,000 people in the last decade has been related to opioid use and abuse, with a 3,000 percent increase in the cost of medical care associated with opioid abuse over the same period.

Current Remedies

While antidepressants and benzodiazepines such as Xanax® and Valium® are used for stress and stress-induced conditions, including anxiety (see "Stress," page 136), one focused antianxiety medication, Buspar®, is chemically unrelated to any benzodiazepines or other sedative pharmaceuticals. Its focus is on the body—treating tension, dizziness, racing heartbeat, and other physical manifestations of anxiety. However, it may take as long as three weeks for the drug to actually ease anxiety symptoms, and even then it may not control them as successfully as benzodiazepine sedatives. While Buspar is not addictive—a plus—it is not valued as a long-term remedy; doctors typically prescribe it for no more than four weeks of use. For anxiety that accompanies withdrawal from opioids, methadone and Suboxone are available, but strict government regulations make them hard to obtain. Suboxone is heavily regulated. Doctors who prescribe the medication are allowed to write only a small number of prescriptions per month.

Why CBD or Medical Cannabis Might Be the Answer

Cannabis was the focus of a study published in *Tidsskrift for den Norske Legeforening* (the *Journal of the Norwegian Medical Association*) in 2010. Researchers found that young adults using cannabis reported a higher level of anxiety and higher rates of prescription drug treatment for their anxiety with sedating benzodiazepines. Researchers initially concluded that young people who use cannabis may be seeking other prescription drugs to enhance the euphoria they experience from cannabis. However, the use of prescription drugs like Valium, Ativan®, or Xanax may be further evidence that young people with anxiety and stress may still go undertreated by the usual medical models and need to seek powerful alternate treatments like cannabis for control of their condition.

Results of a Dutch study, reported in a 2017 edition of the journal *Cannabis and Cannabidiol Research*, indicated that human subjects had lower levels of anxiety and confusion and increased alertness, tranquility, and confidence after using CBD.

Opioid users experiencing cravings and anxiety as they withdrew from addictive drugs were treated with doses of 400mg or 800mg of CBD during studies at New York City's Mount Sinai Hospital. Both doses of CBD were shown to be effective in reducing the desire to use heroin as well as alleviating the anxiety that accompanies acute heroin withdrawal. (See also "Addiction and Withdrawal," page 46.)

Research shows that when using cannabis to treat any kind of anxiety disorder, dosing according to product type is key. CBD appears to ease anxiety at both lower and higher dosing levels. However, THC-rich products have been shown to decrease anxiety levels up to a point and then actually increase them when dosing becomes too high. That's why careful guidance from a professional is vital.

SUPPORTING RESEARCH

A 2016 study, reported in the journal *Psychopharmacology*, notes that a decrease in AEA (arachidonoylethanolamine), a key ECS (endocannabinoid system) chemical, appears to contribute to anxiety as a stress response. But caring for the ECS with regular sleep, healthy diet, exercise, and cannabinoids helps the brain act as a buffer against anxiety and other stress responses. All of these promote balance and homeostasis in the ECS, whose receptors are prominent in the brain. Cannabinoids help shore up the ECS and keep it running smoothly.

For general anxiety, CBD works, as it does with stress, by helping 5-HT1A receptors in the brain release calming serotonin and dopamine. Two terpenes in the hemp plant support that action. Also, limonene, a terpene found in the rind of citrus fruits that is responsible for their scent, is known to improve mood, and linalool, a component of lavender, is hailed as a stress reliever and anxiety calmer. In patients with seasonal affective disorder (SAD), CBD has been shown to induce a significant decrease in anxiety by affecting parts of the brain, including the amygdala and hippocampus, which are linked to episodes of anxiety.

"As far back as I can remember I've had panic reactions in certain situations. Around the age of 22, someone close to me went through a horrible tragedy, and I suffered a complete breakdown. In order to regain control I was put on an anxiety medication. Over the next decade I would be prescribed seven different anxiety medications, with brutal side effects, and without improvement in my symptoms. I had used cannabis as a kid once or twice, and after a second breakdown in my late twenties, I decided to try to save myself another hospital stay by using it again. I found that I had totally misjudged this plant and medical marijuana as some happy-hippie nonsense. My anxiety stopped almost instantly."

—Steve, 38, Manager

Integrative Tip >>>>>

Dr. Zielinski, who specializes in aromatherapy, says: I have come to appreciate that the easiest and, arguably, the most effective approach to successfully manage stress and anxiety is to tap into the power of your olfactory system [sense of smell], because it directly impacts your limbic system—the part of your brain where mood and memories are regulated. Try making these diffuser blends before you go to bed:

- 2 drops ylang-ylang, 1 drop bergamot, 1 drop lavender, 1 drop sweet marjoram, 1 drop Roman chamomile, and 1 drop valerian

- 2 drops lavender, 1 drop clary sage, 1 drop ylang-ylang, and 1 drop vanilla absolute

- 2 drops geranium, 1 drop sweet marjoram, 1 drop patchouli, and 1 drop sweet orange

- 2 drops Roman chamomile, 1 drop rose, and 1 drop palmarosa

NOTE: Use these essential oil diffuser blends according to the manufacturer's instructions, which vary, depending on the product.

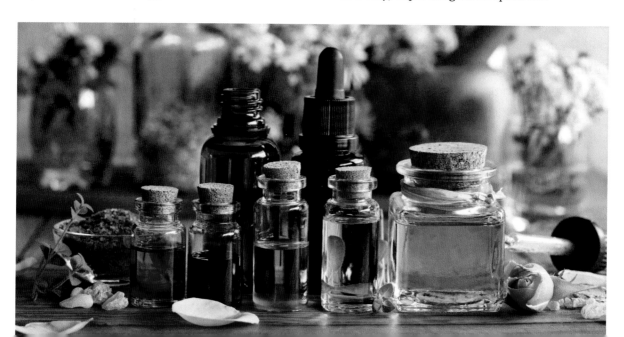

6) Autism Spectrum Disorder

Autism spectrum disorder (ASD) often goes undiagnosed, making the quality of life difficult for thousands of children. A 2020 report from the Autism Research Institute notes that 25 percent of children under the age of eight who have autism spectrum disorder do not find out they have the condition until they're much older—and most of those children are Black or Hispanic. Many conditions go undiagnosed in minority populations, likely related to language barriers and systemic racism. Fortunately, there is growing awareness of ASD and treatment for the condition. ASD is called a developmental disorder because the symptoms appear in a child's first two years and generally continue throughout life. It is also called a spectrum disorder because of the wide range of symptoms and varying degrees of severity of those symptoms. ASD is the umbrella term for three levels of autism determined by the American Psychiatric Association. Mild conditions, or level 1, include Asperger's syndrome, in which children are often gifted, perhaps excelling in math or science, but may lack empathy and social skills. More severe disorders, levels 2 and 3, may cause a child to throw tantrums, be hyperactive, or self-injure. Symptoms may include repetitive behavior; difficulty changing routine; concentrated focus on specific topics, numbers, or details; and sensitivity to light, noise, or smell. While the exact cause of ASD is unknown, risk factors include older parents; a sibling with autism; poor maternal nutrition during pregnancy (especially a lack of folic and fatty acids); low birth weight; exposure to environmental toxins during pregnancy; or chromosomal abnormalities, such as Down syndrome. Experts say that parents can play a critical role in diagnosing their own children, as early as six months, by paying close attention to any sensory, motor, or, later, social and language concerns—and reporting such to their physician. Early diagnosis leads to optimal treatment for children, including managing difficult behaviors and learning new skills while capitalizing on often unique and wondrous strengths.

Current Remedies

Because early detection is on the front line of treatment for ASD, the American Academy of Pediatrics (AAP) recommends that all children be screened for developmental delays starting with their 9-month well-child appointment and for autism starting with their 18-month visit. Therapy, such as helping a child manage and control their behavior within accepted societal rules and learn new skills, is key. There are no specific medications for autism, but several drugs that are used for other conditions are being considered or used for treatment of ASD. These include naltrexone, which is FDA-approved for treating addiction and may help ease repetitive or self-harm behaviors associated with ASD. Attention deficit/hyperactivity disorder (ADHD) medications, such as Ritalin, may help control hyperactivity and focus concentration.

SSRIs (selective serotonin reuptake inhibitors), a class of medications used to treat anxiety, such as fluoxetine, may also be useful.

A great resource for parents and caregivers of people suffering with ASD is the Autism Research Institute, which shares more than 40 years' worth of parent rankings of medicines, therapies, and diets they've found effective.

Why CBD or Medical Cannabis Might Be the Answer

A 2019 study published in *Scientific Reports* and coauthored by Raphael Mechoulam, a groundbreaking Israeli cannabis scientist, has raised hopes for cannabis as a future treatment for ASD. Over a two-year period, 188 patients in the study were treated mainly with an oil containing 30 percent CBD and 1.5 percent THC. After six months of treatment, 83 percent of the participants reported significant or moderate improvement in stress, anxiety, disruptive behavior, and other symptoms of autism. Still, the team underscored that while many patients with autism are being treated with cannabis, "There is a significant lack of knowledge regarding the safety profile and specific symptoms likely to improve under cannabis treatment."

Because the implications of using cannabis to treat autism are still unknown, further research is needed to evaluate the risks versus the gains. The medical community is unsure if cannabis used for medicinal purposes has a different effect on the developing brain than cannabis used for recreational purposes. Clearly, many medications used for the treatment of adolescent psychiatric disorders have the potential to impact the developing brain over the long term, so it's unclear if the effects of cannabis are better or worse. However, cannabis may increase sociability, heighten perception, give a sensation of slowing time, decrease aggression, and increase appetite. Many of these effects, especially as far as increased sociability and decreased aggression are concerned, may be particularly helpful when working with ASD.

Cannabis use does not appear to affect IQ negatively or positively, but it does have other negative outcomes, such as short-term decreases in working memory and in sustained attention and motor coordination. When cannabis is used in the adolescent population, there are potential long-term negative effects on brain development that result in poor educational outcomes, not to mention a heightened risk of addiction. These diminished life achievements have also been associated with an increased risk of psychoses and other chronic mental disorders. Again, we still don't know if cannabis users are driven to use these formulations to self-treat underlying undiagnosed psychiatric conditions. Are the risks associated with cannabis different from the risks associated with multiple prescription antidepressants and antipsychotics administered to young adults with developing brains? We just don't know yet. Further study is desperately needed.

If you plan to work with a physician to administer cannabis to a child or any other patient who has been diagnosed with autism, read this carefully: Legal use of cannabis under the age of 21 varies from state to state, and certain criteria must be met. These include the presence of a debilitating medical condition, a designated caregiver to provide supervision, and an attending physician's statement that verifies the underlying diagnosis of the condition and also certifies that the use of cannabis may mitigate the associated symptoms. The clinician must consider the family's perspective in discussions about the risks and benefits of any treatment that involves the use of cannabis. Clinicians should enter into an agreement with the family to monitor efficacy and safety in a systematic way. Families should be provided with contact information for poison control centers in case of adverse effects or accidental ingestion of cannabis by other family members, and the family should also be counseled about any potential legal implications of using cannabis for therapeutic reasons.

SUPPORTING RESEARCH

If cannabis can indeed ease the various symptoms of autism—including stress, anxiety, and hyperactivity—it is because cannabis interacts with cannabinoid receptors in the ECS (endocannabinoid system), just as it does for those other conditions such as insomnia, anxiety, and pain. Research in a 2015 issue of the journal *Neurotherapeutics* suggests that ECS receptors play a vital role in brain development, reward response, circadian rhythm, and anxiety—all of which are disrupted or imbalanced in autism. The interaction of THC—and also CBD—with these receptors may bring positive results—and hope. A 2017 issue of the *Journal of Pediatric Pharmacology and Therapeutics* notes that the ability of CBD to calm epilepsy could make it a prime candidate for treating similar symptoms in autism. (See also "ADHD," page 49; "Anxiety," page 53; "Depression," page 70; "Epilepsy and Seizures," page 80; "Insomnia," page 101; and "Stress," page 136.)

A NOTE FROM DR. MARY

The use of cannabis by adolescents and young adults is highly controversial and not an accepted practice by most medical organizations. However, the American College of Pediatrics states that if a child is experiencing a life-threatening or debilitating medical condition that cannot be completely controlled by Western medical interventions, the use of cannabis formulations may be considered, as long as appropriate safety precautions are in place. Parents and guardians must work closely with a qualified provider in these circumstances. When using cannabinoid formulations in young adults, studies primarily support the use of tinctures high in CBD with low levels of THC.

"I have seen amazing results from medical use of cannabis. My daughter was diagnosed five years ago with autism, and she has run the gamut of treatments—some successful and some not so successful. I heard about the medical uses of cannabis at a conference and thought, What does cannabis have to do with autism? My daughter is nonverbal and still in diapers and she is seven years old. But now, as a result of treatments with cannabis, her scratching, biting, and tantrums are less frequent. She's much calmer. She has also completely stopped hitting herself in the head."

—Charlotte, 34, Influencer

Integrative Tip >>>>>

Parents of children on the spectrum tend to get a lot of unwanted advice. One of the best things a parent can do is to respect other parents who have previously dealt with similar issues. Nobody has the perfect answer for your child, but it's important to recognize what has worked for other parents—they might have a valuable tip or two.

Elisa Song, MD

Providing integrative care for children with complex medical issues is Dr. Elisa Song's calling. Her patients include those with autism, ADHD, asthma, autoimmune illness, eczema, failure to thrive, food allergies/sensitivities, gastroesophageal reflux disease (GERD), inflammatory bowel disease and other gastrointestinal disorders, seizures and other neurological disorders, and environmental illness. In addition to earning a medical degree from New York University School of Medicine and getting her training in pediatrics at University of California–San Francisco Medical Center, Dr. Song is a student of functional medicine/holistic nutrition, homeopathy, homeopathic detoxification, acupuncture, herbal medicine, and flower essences. She applies all that knowledge to help her patients gain every possible benefit from a holistic healing approach.

7) Brain Health

What is a healthy brain? Is it one that helps you discover and understand the world? Does it guide you reliably through daily tasks and challenges? Is it one that brings purpose and well-being to your life? The National Institute on Aging (NIA) at the National Institutes of Health (NIH) says that all the above describe a healthy brain, along with the ability to remember, learn, plan, concentrate, manage information, and maintain logic, judgment, perspective, and wisdom. Simply put, the NIA states, "Brain health is all about making the most of your brain and helping reduce some risks to it as you age."

The specter of developing dementia is among the greatest fears of people as they age—and with good reason. The Centers for Disease Control and Prevention (CDC) estimates that the risk of Alzheimer's disease—the most common type of dementia—doubles every five years as a person lives beyond age 65. By age 85, some 25–50 percent of the population shows signs of the disease.

Dementia is not a normal age change. It's a disease marked by gradual deterioration of memory, problem-solving, and performance of daily tasks. Another iteration of dementia—vascular dementia—occurs when blood clots in brain arteries destroy small areas of tissue. There is reason to take heart, however: While experts may not know all the reasons for dementia, they do know that it is often connected to things we

can control, such as a stressful, low-activity lifestyle; lack of sleep; and a diet high in sugars and trans fats.

Having said that, there are, unfortunately, unavoidable brain challenges that range from annoying to life-threatening. For instance, a woman going through menopause will likely experience brain fog; that is, a dip in cognitive function. Thankfully the condition is temporary, and sharpness returns when menopause is over. A traumatic physical incident, such as an accident or a war injury, however, may damage parts of the brain and bring deep, long-lasting illness. Emotional trauma, perhaps from war or abuse, may trigger ongoing anxiety, including PTSD (post-traumatic stress disorder). Maintaining a healthy brain will help you navigate these difficult events, and with additional therapy provided by an in-person therapist or through prescriptions or natural medicinals, you can emerge from the fray with all your brain functions intact.

Stroke is a silent killer. Every year it strikes 795,000 people across the United States. In fact, a stroke happens every 40 seconds. Stroke is most often caused by a plaque—a fatty buildup—in an artery that supplies blood to the brain. Gradually the plaque builds and blocks 50 percent and then up to 85 percent of the artery; at that point, the plaque can become irritated and inflamed, injuring the blood vessel. Blood platelets—whose role is to clot a bleeding area—pile up on the plaque in order to control the inflammation. Instead of helping, however, the platelet pileup eventually blocks 100 percent of the artery. That's when blood flow to the brain abruptly stops and a stroke occurs.

Although the unfortunate reality is that 140,000 people in the United States die every year from stroke, 655,000 others recover. However, survivors can be left with weakness, slurred speech, and impaired cognition for the rest of their lives. Stroke has become the leading cause of long-term disability in the United States, in part because many stroke patients have serious long-term side effects and limited access to rehabilitation. Actions we take for granted, like carrying on a conversation or removing a teakettle from the stove, are challenging for stroke patients, making an independent lifestyle impossible. Rehabilitation centers go a long way toward helping patients regain independence. However, stroke prevention is key.

Current Remedies

Exercise has been shown to increase blood flow to the brain, reduce the risk of cardiovascular disease and stroke, promote socializing, and boost production of antioxidants, which protect brain cells—all of which make exercise particularly important for seniors. How much exercise is enough? Not very much, as it turns out. A 2018 NIH-funded study measured how much exercise it takes to boost memory. After 36 healthy young adults pedaled a stationary bike for just 10 minutes at low intensity, their brain's hippocampus—which

is primarily associated with memory—was more active, and links were stronger between the hippocampus and the cerebral cortex, which controls higher functions like thinking and speaking as well as memory. What was the result of those 10 minutes of low-intensity exercise? Improved memory. Surprisingly, more intensive exercise didn't offer more benefit. The message may be this: Treat your body kindly and there's a greater chance your brain will join the party.

Other than exercise, we recommend this plan to help keep your brain in shape:

- Sleep deeply and for as long as you can, for at least seven hours, and for some adults nine or more, to allow your brain to consolidate newly acquired memories.

- Avoid stress, which damages the hippocampus.

- Learn new skills to build cognitive reserve (resistance to brain damage from environmental factors).

- Stay connected, because lonely souls are more at risk for dementia.

- Energize your spirit through meditation and prayer—it has been shown that both practices improve cognitive function.

- Choose a diet that includes brain-boosting omega-3s, found in salmon and almonds, to help protect brain cells.

- Watch your salt and, especially, your sugar intake. Too much sugar leads to inflammation and a buildup of the protein beta amyloid, which, when it accumulates in the brain, can lead to Alzheimer's disease. High glucose also damages arteries and can cause stroke.

Ongoing moderate exercise and a diet low in sugar and fat will go marathon miles toward protecting your brain against stroke. But if stroke or another traumatic brain injury does occur, wide-ranging physical, psychological, and emotional rehabilitative therapies are available. In addition, medications may be prescribed for the anxiety, pain, and even psychosis that may accompany those conditions.

Why CBD or Medical Cannabis Might Be the Answer

In a 2017 study, reported in the journal *Frontiers of Pharmacology*, adult patients with a number of non–brain-related medical conditions underwent three months of treatment with cannabis. All the patients improved in performance of routine tasks, and researchers saw changes in brain activation patterns in the prefrontal cortex: The brains of study participants actually appeared similar to those of healthy participants in the control [the untreated group]. At the end of the study patients also reported that their primary health concerns had seen improvement, including a decrease in use of opioids, benzodiazepines, anti-depressants, and other prescription medications.

If you heard, as a young adult, that you would become a pothead or fry your brain if you smoked cannabis, that's because some early studies supported that theory. One of them, a population-based New Zealand study, published in a 2012 edition of the journal *Proceedings of the National Academy of Sciences* (*PNAS*), followed 1,037 patients for 38 years and suggested that cannabis users saw a six-point decline in IQ. This initial study was worrisome. However, in 2016, a somewhat larger study in the United Kingdom that followed 2,235 patients since 1991 showed no association between young adult or adolescent cannabis use and any changes in IQ.

Finally, in 2016, a 20-year study in the United States of 3,066 people, who used cannabis over that period, really sealed the deal: It found *absolutely* no relationship between lower IQ and cannabis use. The US study was particularly convincing because it included 47 pairs of discordant identical twins; that is, one twin in each pair smoked cannabis, and one did not. That data is compelling because the twins were identical, DNA-wise, and presumably much of their childhood was similar.

We can make a very good argument that if there was no significant difference among the 3,066 people in the study, 47 pairs of whom were discordant identical twins, then we can be reasonably assured that there is no significant effect of cannabis use on IQ. However, some studies show a decrease in short-term memory with heavy use of cannabis. But even among those users, normal memory is restored within just three months, and in some cases in as little as three days, with the cessation of cannabis use.

A 2017 study in the journal *Frontiers in Pharmacology* indicates that using cannabis is more beneficial to an older person's more fully developed brain. Since older adults are most at risk for stroke, is it possible they could benefit from cannabinoids to help prevent stroke? Maybe. One study, published in Japan, reported potential improvements in a patient's ability to ward off stroke when using CBD. And an increasing number of publications are focusing on CBD's neuroprotective, anti-inflammatory, and antioxidant benefits—not only to protect from ischemic (blood clot–related) stroke but also from chronic diseases of the central nervous system, such as Alzheimer's, Parkinson's, and multiple sclerosis. It's important to clarify that most of what we know about CBD in relation to stroke is based only on laboratory experiments. Researchers are learning about the effect of cannabinoids in test tubes in the laboratory and may never conduct large, human population–based studies. Some researchers are examining patient records and making correlations between variables—that is, among people who consumed cannabinoid formulations and those who didn't—in order to devise formulations that could help people with a variety of conditions.

SUPPORTING RESEARCH

Researchers are finding that, rather than interacting with CB1 and CB2 receptors, which affect our health, CBD and other cannabinoids may be beneficial in boosting brain health. These phyto-cannabinoids, which are both anti-inflammatory and antioxidant, carry inherent neuroprotectant properties that could help guard brain cells from long-term degeneration and damage from environmental toxins.

The 2017 study in *Frontiers in Pharmacology*, noted previously, also showed that THC may be able to boost cognitive function. That boost might be explained through studies carried out with mature mice. When given low doses of THC, their cognitive decline was reversed, perhaps because the aging endocannabinoid system gets a boost, or upregulation, from the increased signaling prompted by the THC. Researchers found, however, that the same amount of THC given to young mice resulted in lowered cognition. Researchers are continuing to study the potentially positive impact of THC on boosting brain health in aging populations.

Research shows that CBD may or may not act through the endocannabinoid system, but it appears to be working to support healthy brain function through other mechanisms besides the CB receptors—and since 2018, scientists have been looking for the operative mechanism. As with Parkinson's (see page 125), NIH-supported studies in 2012 and 2014 showed that CBD helped reverse cognitive decline in rats that had been treated with iron—a mineral known for triggering memory loss and that is present in the brains of Alzheimer's sufferers. CBD also helped clean out proteins and other particles that can accumulate and trigger cell death in the brains of patients suffering from Alzheimer's.

As far as stroke prevention is concerned, ongoing studies show that CBD helps reduce heart rate and high blood pressure, which contribute to stroke. One study using mice concluded that CBD helps blood vessels relax and increase in diameter, so that blood can actually flow around plaque blockages. If a stroke occurs, quick administration of CBD may help increase cerebral blood flow during the stroke and immediately afterward—to potentially help minimize damage to brain tissue. Early laboratory data also suggests that cannabinoids can contribute to the development of new nerve growth, or neuroregeneration, so stay tuned! Early studies and animal models focused on the use of cannabinoids to potentially help victims of stroke look promising.

❝My dad lived an amazing life. He was in World War II and had combat experience. He returned from the war and built a successful business in mechanics. But a diagnosis of Alzheimer's a few years before his death left him initially with memory loss that was subsequently followed by increasing agitation, and I was surprised by his aggression. He also started to relive memories from the war, which he had tried so hard to suppress for such a long time. Someone suggested we try medical cannabis. The first night after using it, my father slept through the night for the first time in weeks. It improved the quality of his life during that difficult time.❞

—Ellie, 62, Interior Designer

Dr. Christine Schaffner

Dr. Christine Schaffner is a board-certified naturopathic physician and graduate of Bastyr University in Washington State. She completed her undergraduate studies in pre-medicine and psychology at the University of Virginia in Charlottesville. Dr. Schaffner's style of practice is rooted in traditional naturopathic principles. She believes in the importance of establishing a strong foundation to achieve optimal health. Dr. Schaffner combines both naturopathic and conventional therapies to develop individualized treatment plans that focus on addressing the underlying cause of complex chronic illness. Dr. Schaffner is an expert in the glymphatic system, the immune system of the central nervous system that controls inflammation and promotes brain health and healing.

Integrative Tip >>>>>

Your immune system responds to experiences, and your brain has a hard time differentiating between what you watch on television and real-life experiences. Take some time today to consider the inputs you are giving your brain through television programs. While you may consider what you view on television as entertainment or simply as a way to pass the time, your brain may be registering the experience as a series of traumas from visual and auditory inputs that stimulate traumatic responses rather than relaxation. Providing your brain with interesting and thought-provoking programs, instead of sensationalized entertainment, could support healthier brain activity over your lifetime.

8) Cancer

Cancer treatment holds a very special place in my heart and probably in yours, too. I'm sure that many people who are reading this book or who are involved in medical cannabis are either personally dealing with cancer or know someone who has been impacted by it.

Cancer—known by ancients as "the crab" for its spreading, crablike shape as it invades the body—is the number two killer after heart disease in America. The risk of dying from cancer is more than 22 percent for men and more than 18 percent for women in the United States. Of the more than 100 kinds of cancer, the most common is breast cancer—with 271,270 new cases

in 2019 in the United States—followed by lung, prostate, and colorectal cancers. Laryngeal and lung cancers have the lowest survival rates. In some cases cancer is inherited, but most kinds are prompted by three main—and preventable—environmental factors: smoking, pollutants like radiation and factory toxins, and poor diet and obesity. Alcoholism and lack of sleep are also risk factors. Eighty percent of cancer cases take hold in people over the age of 55, likely due to an accumulation of factors over the years. As a side note, Kentucky has the highest cancer rate in the country.

The start of any cancer begins with cells that have gone awry. The trillions of cells that comprise your body are all part of a well-honed system: They generate, flourish, divide, and die on schedule, with new cells taking their place. Sometimes that mechanism goes haywire. Cells proliferate, crowd out normal cells, live too long, and form cancerous tumors that can metastasize (spread throughout the body).

In 2020, more than 1.8 million cases of cancer across the nation will likely be diagnosed with some 606,520 deaths, according to the American Cancer Society. But there is some good news: While cancer deaths peaked in the 1990s, as of 2017, there has been a 30 percent decline in US deaths—3 million fewer—largely attributed to campaigns against smoking. Other statistics bring hope, too: Some 16 million cancer survivors are thriving today, and their numbers are on the rise. Unlike other conditions that have a beginning and an end, however, cancer is never fully cured, but it *can* go into remission for decades, thanks to rapidly growing treatments: precision surgery using robots, bone marrow transplants, cryoablation (the use of an extremely cold liquid or instrument used to freeze and destroy abnormal tissue), along with personalized chemotherapy regimens. For survivors, remission is a new chance at life.

Current Treatments

Depending on the kind of cancer and its stage, a doctor may direct a patient to any number of therapies. Surgery may be used to remove a contained tumor (where cancer hasn't spread to the surrounding tissue) with a robotic arm, which offers precision, flexibility, fewer complications, and more rapid recovery.

In radiation therapy, beams of energy from high-powered machines shrink a tumor by destroying the genetic matter that controls the makeup and division of cells. While X-rays are the most common kind of radiation therapy, newer proton therapy is giving surgeons more control and leaving patients with fewer side effects.

Cryoablation, sometimes used in cervical, bone, prostate, and eye cancers, where surgeries are difficult, involves injecting an extremely cold gas directly into cancer cells to kill them. It is also a pain therapy for cancers that have metastasized.

Chemotherapy may be best known: A powerful chemical cocktail kills fast-growing cancer cells either in a single tumor or a bodywide metastasis. Mixtures differ based on the kind of cancer being treated. Chemotherapy can be administered by mouth in a liquid or pill form, by injection or infusion, or topically. Like radiation, chemotherapy comes with side effects such as nausea, vomiting, diarrhea, hair loss, and fatigue.

Why CBD or Medical Cannabis Might Be the Answer

When oncologists are thinking about making informed decisions about cannabis for their patients, only 30 percent feel they can advise their patients about cannabinoid formulations. Over 70 percent of oncologists feel that cannabis has value in cancer treatment, especially in the area of symptom management, but fewer than 30 percent actually feel comfortable helping patients make an informed decision about how to use cannabinoid formulations; they still have a long way to go before they will even talk about cannabis as a treatment, but I think that's just fine. Your primary care physician can always refer you to a specialist when questions or problems fall outside their own area of expertise.

There are various suspected mechanisms for how cannabis—especially from plant-derived phytocannabinoids—can affect potential tumor activity. There are also multiple different cannabinoids, including THC, CBN, CBD, and CBL, as well as a number of synthetic cannabinoids, such as WIN 55,212-2, that are the focus of research. We still don't know for sure which cannabinoids are the strongest cancer fighters and which ones work best alone or in combination, but scientists are working hard to determine the most effective ratios for cancer treatment.

Cancer patients endure significant side effects while they undergo chemotherapy. We have to remember that cannabis first came to light in cancer treatment because of its beneficial effects in reducing chemotherapy-induced nausea and vomiting. Those benefits have been supported by several long-term and conclusive trials. The benefits of using cannabis products to reduce pain associated with chemotherapy were put to the test in 28 randomized controlled trials, and expert panelists (all independent specialists) concluded that there is moderate quality evidence to bolster this contention. So we can support the use of cannabis in pain treatments for chemotherapy patients, but we still need more studies to figure out which formulations in what ratios would be ideal as pain treatments for chemotherapy patients.

In addition, several smaller studies have suggested that adding cannabis to some chemotherapy treatments could reduce the toxic effects of chemotherapy on the nervous system and heart, by lowering the incidence of painful neuropathies and heart conditions experienced by so many patients after cancer treatments.

It's important to note that cannabinoid formulations should not be used *instead of* other chemotherapies. The American Cancer Society and most oncologists do not recommend forgoing conventional therapy in favor of using only cannabis products. However, a number of well-informed doctors recommend using cannabis *in addition to* chemotherapy for cancer, in some cases, to add to its effectiveness and to control related symptoms.

SUPPORTING RESEARCH

There are a number of different ways in which cannabis products work to fight cancer independent of other chemotherapies. One of the most fascinating mechanisms is the PGP (P-glycoprotein) pump—a protein in the cell membrane that "pumps" toxins out of cells. PGP pumps also happen to recognize beneficial chemotherapy drugs as toxins. Since PGP pumps work to remove toxins, they pump chemotherapy chemicals out of the cells to help protect the cells from the toxic chemotherapy. This prevents the drugs from exerting their healing effects. Because of PGP pump action, many cancer cells become increasingly resistant to anticancer therapy, especially as the cells get more and more exposure to chemotherapy. PGP pumps are considered one of the main contributors to the development of resistance to chemotherapy. CBD appears to inhibit the action of PGP pumps; thus, CBD could potentially improve the effectiveness of chemotherapy by allowing the chemotherapy to remain in the cancer cell longer and destroy more cancer cells.

The data about cannabis and cancer is encouraging and exciting, but it is important to be aware that the data has been obtained from a laboratory; that is, from a test tube or a petri dish. It was not derived from individual cancer patients except in some unusual cases, which we describe shortly. With that in mind, here are some other ways that cannabis might benefit cancer treatment.

Cannabis appears to work against cancer by stimulating the immune system to kill cancer at "security checkpoints." That action is the responsibility of the T cells—special cells in the immune system that detect normal versus abnormal proteins as part of their usual body-scanning process. When unwanted cells are detected, T cells set to work to harness the immune system and enhance antitumor responses, such as delaying tumor growth and rejecting tumors altogether.

Cannabis also has potential benefits in helping cancer cells recognize their mutant character and proceed to natural cell death. Cancer cells do not perceive themselves as ordinary cells that age and die. Instead, they act and become immortal. Helping cancer cells move through a normal process of cell death, or apoptosis, is a focus of cancer research. Cannabis appears to interact with signaling pathways that prompt normal cell proliferation, survival, and eventually death. By stimulating the CB receptors, cannabis triggers processes that help cells recognize when they're ready to die.

Cannabis can also stimulate antioxidant activity to help fight cancer by protecting cells. In addition, cannabis boosts a special tissue-supporting protein called TIMP-1, which blocks toxic enzymes from invading healthy cells, thus boosting normal cell proliferation and guiding cells toward natural apoptosis.

Finally, researchers have discovered that cannabis can promote a more robust response to chemotherapy (as opposed to not using cannabis at all in conjunction with chemotherapy). This is the case especially when cannabis is administered before chemotherapy begins. In a study of brain cancer, using mice, cannabis was found to boost the effects of radiation therapy. Cannabinoids have also been shown to enhance the chemotherapy medication paclitaxel (Taxol®) in fighting gastric carcinomas. When cannabinoids were administered with dangerous chemotherapeutic agents like gemcitabine, the plant-drug synergy was shown to inhibit pancreatic adenocarcinoma cell growth. And cannabis has been shown to boost chemotherapy's potency in treating certain leukemias.

" *I was in and out of the hospital with weight loss and stomach pain. The doctors thought I had an ulcer. Eventually, I was diagnosed with ovarian cancer. I was told that I would have six weeks to live without treatment. The cancer had spread to my small intestine, and there were spots in my stomach where cancer had been detected as well. I went on chemotherapy and got sepsis from a catheter. The first time I tried cannabis to help with the side effects of chemo, I was giggly and tired but not at all aggressive. I use it at night to control the side effects. Now, all of my tumors are gone except for just a little bit in my stomach.* **"**

—**Melanie, 51, College Professor**

Integrative Tip > > > > >
Make smart choices when buying and preparing meats. According to the United States Department of Agriculture, processed meats—such as bacon, sausage, luncheon meats, and hot dogs—contain nitrates, which increase the risk of colorectal cancers. Steer clear of charbroiling and deep-frying, which create cancer-causing substances. Instead, sauté meat in a little olive oil or bake it with vegetable broth for moisture, and poach fish.

9) Depression

Depression is debilitating. And isolating. While a person suffers from it, loved ones struggle to understand the deep sadness and feelings of uselessness and guilt that sentence that person to days and weeks of curling up in a fetal position under the bedcovers. When depression is at work, a once-joyful individual no longer finds pleasure in everyday activities, thought processes are impaired, and decision making is irrational. In addition, sleeplessness is an issue that aggravates the condition. Sudden trauma or personal loss, a change in hormonal balance (due to pregnancy or menopause), a chronic disease that shows no signs of healing, or possibly a change in a person's brain chemistry are just a few of the triggers for depression.

There are many natural remedies for depression, however, including exercise, as simple as walking; a mood-enhancing diet, rich in brain-boosting omega-3 fatty acids; eight hours of uninterrupted sleep; and conversation with a beloved family member or friend. But sometimes our actions are not rational and our behavior

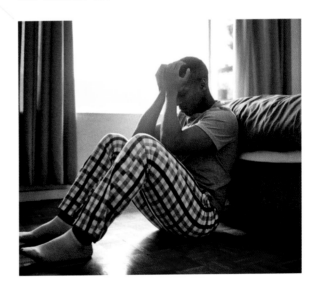

cycles between extremes; that is, "I'm better," "I'm not better." Repeat. As of 2020, the NIMH (National Institute of Mental Health) estimates that 16.2 million American adults—6.7 percent of the adult population—have at least one major depressive episode in a year. And about 1.5 percent of the adult population—more women than men—experience dysthymia, a chronic, low-grade form of depression that can last for months or years. Depression is a serious condition that demands treatment. Fortunately, hopeful discoveries in cannabis treatment are on the horizon.

Current Remedies

While antidepressants that include selective serotonin reuptake inhibitors (SSRIs), such as Paxil® and Prozac®, are generally prescribed as first responders for cases of depression, they may bring a patient close to remission and then fall short. It is only a matter of time until symptoms recur and a cyclical pattern of relapse and remission takes hold. In some cases of depression, a person's genetic code may be responsible for the condition. For instance, researchers have found that the gene of the cannabinoid receptor CNR1 can have polymorphisms, or variations, that make a person more vulnerable both to developing depression after a traumatic life event and also to developing resistance to antidepressants used to treat the condition.

Aside from prescription medicines, exciting new studies are taking place with psilocybin, the compound found in what is known as magic mushrooms. While psilocybin is hallucinogenic in its raw form, it is a depression fighter when used as a controlled medicine. A single dose has been shown to reduce the symptoms of depression for many, many months. Scientists are experimenting with ways to produce medical psilocybin by extracting its DNA from mushrooms and then inserting it into E. coli—the common bacterium found in your gut. As the E. coli multiplies, the presence of the psilocybin increases in stable, regulated, controlled ways. Such controlled bioproduction of psilocybin will allow us to move forward aggressively with clinical trials for this very hopeful depression fighter.

Why CBD or Medical Cannabis
Might Be the Answer

People have long used cannabis to lift mood. That's 3,000 years of "long." In the 21st century, studies have backed up that time-honored usage. A cross-sectional study—that is, an analysis of data across a sample population—demonstrated that people who use cannabis on an occasional-to-daily basis may be less depressed than those who have never consumed the plant. And the results of seven other cross-sectional studies, noted in a 2017 issue of the journal *Clinical Psychology Review*, gave clear evidence that medical cannabis raises depressed mood. There is hopeful news, too, for those who suffer from depression triggered by chronic pain. A 2017 study, published in the journal *La Clinica*

Terapeutica, involved 338 patients who reported reductions in pain intensity and disability, as well as reductions in related anxiety and depression. Those results led researchers to suggest that medical marijuana could add significantly to a chronic pain treatment protocol.

SUPPORTING RESEARCH

In recent years, clinical evidence has mounted, linking the development of depression to a low-functioning ECS (endocannabinoid system) and suggesting that addressing that deficit could open the door to revolutionary new treatments. In clinical studies reported in 2018 in the journal *Frontiers in Molecular Neuroscience*, researchers found a lack of healthy 2-AG endocannabinoids circulating in the bodies of women diagnosed with major depression—and whose depression lasted for long periods. Other patients' brains were shown to have underactive CB1R receptors, which normally help keep the calming chemical serotonin circulating in the body. Without sufficient levels of serotonin, anxiety and depression set in. Still other research, as noted previously, showed that a genetic variant of the CNR1 receptor gene increases a person's vulnerability to depression and other mood disorders.

A NOTE FROM DR. MARY

In most cases, strain selection is specific to the individual and their comprehensive collection of medical conditions. However, in the case of treating depression with cannabis, a special mention needs to be made of Harlequin, or Cherry Pie if Harlequin is unavailable. Across my practice, so many patients have reported excellent results with these two strains that they've become my regular recommendation for patients dealing with depression. I always prefer an inhalation method so that the administration amount can be modified based on day-to-day needs.

❝ *At the age of 14, I was diagnosed with a chemical imbalance and clinical depression. I was prescribed an assortment of SSRI drugs for depression and gabapentin for my anxiety/panic attacks. From age 15 to age 30, I consumed about 30 pounds of these prescription drugs. Then I felt inspired to replace the pharmaceuticals with cannabis. My secret has been microdosing THC in the form of vape or edible (5mg) to start the day and 5mg to end the day. I supplement throughout the day with CBD-based vapes that include calming terpenes, such as linalool and myrcene, and mood-enhancing ones, such as limonene and pinene. My morning routine includes breathing exercises, jogging, and listening to uplifting music. April 2020 marked my sixth year without taking any pharmaceutical drugs.* ❞

—Oleg MaryAces, Founder, Lock & Key Remedies, and Cannabis Educator

Oleg MaryAces

Oleg MaryAces entered the cannabis industry in April 2012, with the development of portable vaporizers for use with cannabis extracts. After two years of research and development and after manufacturing the devices in China, Oleg shifted focus to US-based production and collaborated with a Connecticut manufacturer to design a new line of mechanical and electronic vaporizers. Oleg, along with his partners, founded Lock & Key Remedies in November 2016 to develop a line of health and wellness products that incorporate nonintoxicating ingredients extracted from cannabis plants. Oleg is dedicated to educating people about CBD, cannabinoids, terpenes, and how those compounds interact with the endocannabinoid system.

Integrative Tip >>>>>

Adolescents who stand, move, and exercise during the day are less prone to depression in later life, according to a study of 4,257 teens published in a 2020 edition of the journal *Lancet Psychiatry*. The report adds that kids don't have to join a football or tennis team to be active: Even standing up while talking with friends or doing homework counts. Experts recommend that schools integrate movement into the school day through standing or active lessons, such as walking through the woods to identify plants instead of merely looking them up in a botany textbook. At home, parents might consider installing a standing desk for doing homework.

10) Digestive Health

It's a monthly event—and it's not a party! According to the American College of Gastroenterology, heartburn visits some 60 million Americans in any 30-day period. Included in that number are the 15 million who experience it on a daily basis—with pregnant women and the elderly at the top of the list. Officially known as gastroesophageal reflux disease, or GERD, this uncomfortable condition takes place in the esophagus, just steps away from your heart. Symptoms include burning chest pain after eating and when lying prone at night, pain that worsens as you bend over, and a bitter taste in the mouth. If you're suffering from these symptoms and want to understand and address them, start by looking at what causes GERD: The sphincter, the muscle between the esophagus and stomach, becomes lax. Instead of closing off the stomach, where acid breaks down food, it allows a little food and acid to leak upward into the esophagus. That's known as acid reflux. To calm the action, doctors may prescribe medications and recommend lifestyle changes, such as putting the brakes on your

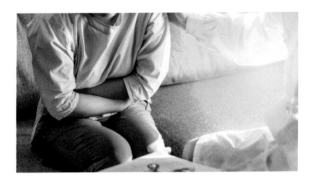

high-stress lifestyle and dropping spicy, heavy and fatty, or caffeine-rich foods.

GERD is just one reason you need to take care of the beautiful, 30-foot-long digestive tract that runs from your mouth all the way to your rectum and that includes your esophagus, stomach, intestines, and related digestive organs like the liver and pancreas. Irritable bowel syndrome (IBS) is another gastrointestinal disorder associated with abdominal pain, often relieved with bowel movements with alternating bouts of diarrhea or constipation. The International Foundation for Gastrointestinal Disorders reports rates of prevalence ranging from 10–15 percent of the population worldwide, with 3.5 million IBS doctor visits a year in the United States alone. One to two people out of every ten experience abdominal pain at least three days a month, changes in stool consistency and frequency, and diarrhea or constipation—or both. Here's the usual backstory for that misery: A hitch in the rhythmic muscular action of the intestines causes basic discomfort, which is then aggravated by spicy foods, lactose or gluten products, and stress. To compound the discomfort, constipation caused by the disorder may also produce hemorrhoids—swollen, painful veins in the anus.

In the case of autoimmune inflammatory bowel diseases (IBDs) like Crohn's disease and ulcerative colitis, the immune system mistakes food and helpful bacteria for toxins and sends white blood cells to destroy them. Abdominal pain, diarrhea, bowel obstruction, and open sores may result.

Current Remedies

To help ease symptoms of GERD and IBS, doctors may prescribe medications and recommend lifestyle changes, such as eliminating spicy foods, alcohol, caffeine, chocolate, and citrus, as well as reducing stress.

For GERD, doctors may prescribe antacids like Rolaids® or Tums® to neutralize stomach acid as short-term remedies; medications called H-2 receptor blockers, like cimetidine (Tagamet®) and famotidine (Pepcid®), provide longer relief and may also help decrease acid production; and proton pump inhibitors—stronger acid blockers, like lansoprazole (Prevacid®) and omeprazole (Prilosec®)—give irritated tissue time to heal.

Depending on the IBS symptoms, a doctor may prescribe fiber supplements or laxatives for constipation; over-the-counter antidiarrheal medications for diarrhea; anticholinergic medications for bowel spasms; and tricyclic antidepressants, which control pain in the intestines and also help with the anxiety and depression that can accompany IBS. For IBD, an immunosuppressant drug, such as azathioprine (including Azasan® and Imuran®), which suppresses the immune response and counters release of inflammatory chemicals may be called for; in the case of Crohn's disease (another IBD), antibiotics may be prescribed to treat infection.

Why CBD or Medical Cannabis Might Be the Answer

Research shows that administering CBD, THC, or a mix of both may provide relief for the diarrheal component of IBS.

For IBD patients suffering from the symptoms of nausea, diarrhea, constipation, and abdominal pain, which is exacerbated by eating, life can be very difficult. So it's not surprising that in a study published in 2013 in the journal *Inflammatory Bowel Disease*, 12.4 percent of 292 inflammatory bowel disease patients reported regular use of cannabis, which seems to help relieve the anxiety and pain surrounding the disorder. Did cannabis also relieve inflammation? Probably.

In a study of 18 patients with ulcerative colitis, colon biopsy tissues were treated with CBD. Results of the study showed a reduction in mast cell number, inducible nitric oxide, and TNF alpha—all inflammatory agents—compared to non–CBD-treated tissues. It appears that CBD works directly on the lining of the colon to reduce inflammation.

If you're dealing with chronic abdominal pain and taking significant immune-modulating medications to ease symptoms, here is news for you: In this same study of patients with ulcerative colitis, 16.4 percent of the participants said that cannabis was "very helpful" for relief of abdominal pain, nausea, and diarrhea. If the patients in that very small and short study derived benefits from using cannabis, it might be worth a try for you. As a result, you may see a reduction in inflammation, as well as experience less anxiety and chronic pain. Cannabis may help give you a good night's sleep, too.

SUPPORTING RESEARCH

In a 2016 issue of the journal *Cannabis and Cannabinoid Research*, neurologist Ethan Russo proposed that IBS may be the result of a deficient endocannabinoid system (ECS), the functioning of which is to maintain homeostasis—that is, balance in your body. Studies for more than a decade have shown that cannabinoids may interact with the ECS to help alleviate the pain and discomfort of IBS and other digestive conditions.

As you'll recall, the ECS is a complex system, comprising receptors (CB1 and CB2) that function much like plant-derived THC and CBD. CB1 receptors are located throughout the lining of the gut, and CB2 receptors are also located in the smooth muscles that control peristalsis, the action of moving food forward as it is digested in the intestine. Research shows that for people who are suffering predominantly from the symptoms of diarrhea and constipation, cannabidiols may interact with CB1 and CB2 receptors to inhibit movement and secretion and regulate the sensation of pain across the gastrointestinal tract. The activation of CB1 receptors could be more helpful in people with diarrhea-predominant IBS because the stimulation of CB1 receptors can slow gut motility.

In a study published in a 2011 issue of *Gastroenterology,* 75 IBS patients who were treated with a synthetic cannabis saw decreased colon motion when they weren't eating, compared to patients who had been given a placebo. Decreased motion of the colon resulted in less diarrhea, and the effects were greatest in IBS patients with diarrhea or diarrhea alternating with constipation. Similar studies of IBS sufferers using cannabinoid formulations also showed lower sensations of pain. So it appears that impacting the cannabinoid system with CBD or THC—or a mix of CBD and THC—may result in improvement in both the diarrhea and abdominal-pain components of IBS.

"*I began using medical cannabis two months ago for my irritable bowel syndrome. It's been a miracle! My IBS pain has been reduced dramatically. I also have chronic neck pain and stiffening that got better, too! Two for one! It took me more time than I expected to adjust the amount so that I wasn't getting high, because I'm not interested in all that. I heartily recommend it.***"**

—Samuel, 45, Clergyman

Dr. Tom O'Bryan

When it comes to getting healthy, Dr. Tom O'Bryan's goal for you is "making it easy to do the right thing." As an internationally recognized speaker on food sensitivities, environmental toxins, and the development of autoimmune disorders such as celiac disease, Dr. O'Bryan tells audiences that identifying the reasons behind a condition leads to finding the best remedy. Dr. O'Bryan is the founder of www.theDr.com and the visionary behind the Gluten Summit: A Grain of Truth, which brings together world-renowned experts to share findings on gluten's connection to diseases and disorders.

Integrative Tip >>>>>

Dr. Mary's favorite secret weapon is cabbage. Cabbage has anticancer properties, it's loaded with fiber to heal your gastrointestinal tract, and is virtually calorie-free. Mary has eaten at least one head of cabbage a week for the last eight years. She uses it in pasta dishes to extend the dish without adding calories, eats it raw in salads and slaws, and puts it in stir-fries and soups. You'll find a place for cabbage everywhere once you start to use it, and you'll be rewarded with a healthier digestive tract. If you're not used to a high-fiber diet, start with cooked cabbage in soups and other dishes before going to raw recipes to help aid in digestion.

11) Elder Care and End of Life

The twilight years are meant to bring joy—retirement, grandchildren, travel. These years also bring the effects of aging—lowered immunity, thinning bone and muscle, hearing loss, and, in some cases, dementia. Our physical bodies wear down under the stress of time. With good health care and a wellness regimen—including healthy diet, plenty of sleep, exercise, and rich social and spiritual connections—joy can be yours for decades. But get ready for bumps in the road, and maybe a hill or two, along the way. Every senior is likely to have at least one condition that's discussed in this book. In any case, their response to that condition should be guided by a trusted family physician and supported by family.

And then there is end of life to consider—a conversation that is relevant for everyone, not only the elderly. Disease or accident can take us at any age, and while extraordinary advancements in medicine can help us sustain life, many choose to proceed with only minimal or no treatment, whether it's surgery, drugs, or other life support. Palliative, or hospice, care is the answer for many, in a setting where the focus is no longer on healing a condition but on managing pain

and bringing emotional, psychological, and spiritual contentment to the patient. Whether in a patient's home, a care facility, a hospital, or an inpatient hospice, a team of medical, social, and spiritual caregivers helps minimize pain and apprehension as the patient moves as serenely as possible through the end stages of life.

Conditions that bring on the end of life may include cancer, congestive heart failure, kidney disease, Parkinson's, Alzheimer's, and traumatic brain injury, among many others. Managing pain is crucial, especially with end-stage cancers. But other physical concerns, like shortness of breath, constipation, and nausea, must be managed, too. Psychological and spiritual concerns are key, as nearing the unknown can bring stress, loneliness, depression, and sleepless nights. Hospice patients often suffer anxiety, as they worry about putting their affairs in order and securing the future of their loved ones.

An excellent palliative care team can help a person feel more in control by listening to personal goals, reviewing treatment options, and keeping team members, family members, and the patient informed along the way. While pain medications are administered, comforting gestures, such as gentle massage, soothing music, and simply holding hands, go a long way toward helping a patient through what can be a beautiful transition.

Current Treatments

For elder care, each treatment depends on the condition and must be carefully discussed with a family health-care expert. For end-of-life palliative care, a number of medications may be given to ease pain and anxiety. A study published by the National Institutes of Health (NIH) reported that acetaminophen is the medication most commonly used to reduce fever and pain. Antispasmodics help relax muscles, and antidepressants and anti-anxiety medications may be prescribed for depression and anxiety. A drug called atropine can help control the production of excess mucus, saliva, and acid. Cancers, which bring excessive pain, are most often treated with fentanyl and morphine. As noted in the official journal of the American Nurses Association, *American Nurse Today*, morphine, which is the preferred pain reliever for cancer, is also used to relieve the sensation of shortness of breath as life comes to a close.

Why CBD or Medical Cannabis Might Be the Answer

If an older patient is considering adding medical marijuana to treatment for chronic pain or cancer, or for any other reason, it might be a good idea. But resistance to the use of medical cannabis is understandable. While cannabis has been available for 4,000 years as a medicinal herb, there has been a lot of controversy surrounding its use in the United States (see page 11).

Since seniors use one-third of all prescription drugs on the market, and those drugs are expensive and fraught with side effects, it might be reasonable to consider CBD or medical marijuana as an alternative. Analysis by the National Institute on Drug Abuse (NIDA) has shown that when medical marijuana is legalized in a state and dispensaries are available, there are fewer deaths by opioids, less treatment with opioids, and a decrease in the number of people who self-report opioid abuse.

The studies that follow showcase the positive impact that medical marijuana or CBD, combined with other treatments, can have on relieving pain, decreasing cancer-related symptoms and side effects, and reducing the need for opioids.

A study of the use and efficacy of medical marijuana among seniors was published in the *European Journal of Internal Medicine* in 2018. In the study, seniors 65 years old and older, who had been getting medical marijuana from a dispensary for at least six months, were given a questionnaire over a two-year period. The participants—2,736 seniors, with an average age of 74—completed the questionnaire. The results were reassuring. A little more than 66 percent of the group reported decreases in pain. Patients reported that their pain level, when rated on a scale of 1 to 10, fell from a 10 to between 8 and 4. In addition, 60.8 percent of cancer patients in the same study reported a reduction in symptoms related to cancer or the side effects of chemotherapy. At six months, 93.7 percent of the patients who filled out the questionnaire reported improvement in their symptoms overall. The most common adverse effects of using medical marijuana—dizziness and dry mouth—were reported in less than 10 percent of the patients. In addition, 18.1 percent of the group had either stopped or significantly reduced their use of opioids.

If you are interested in trying CBD or marijuana for a medical condition but are concerned that you might get high or feel like you're out of control or dissociated (that is, disconnected from the world) in some way, careful titration (gradual dosing) will help, without giving you unwanted side effects. In a report of 3,695 emergency room visits by patients who'd used THC-rich cannabis for recreational consumption and then complained of unwanted side effects, researchers determined that the patients may not have properly calculated how much they had taken and were experiencing the late onset properties of cannabis. In other words, the patients literally enjoyed too much of a good thing; the first dose felt so good that a second was taken in order to feel even better. The result? A dose that delivered anything but the desired effect. Still, the symptoms—elevated heart rate, panic, agitation, and nausea—were not serious and required only symptomatic care. The patients were discharged within eight hours.

The respiratory consequences of inhaling cannabis smoke, on the other hand, can be much more serious for some people. Some 150 compounds come from smoked, burned cannabis, including five polycystic aromatic hydrocarbons—strong carcinogens that include tar and carbon monoxide. Vaporization reduces their formation. So if you're worried about adverse effects from cannabis use,

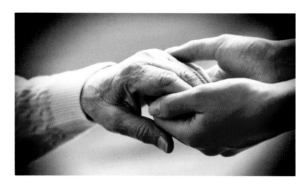

start your dose low, go slow, and consider vaping or using a tincture to avoid the risks of smoke exposure over time.

In a 2017 study published in *Pharmaceutical Journal*, cannabis was reported to be effective in improving quality of life for patients receiving palliative care. Not only did it stimulate their appetite and help them gain weight; it led to better sleep, greater contentment, and more energy as well. Itching and pain were relieved, and opioid use was lower. A 2016 issue of *Current Oncology* reported success in using both CBD and THC with end-stage patients. It eased symptoms of nausea, vomiting, and pain that accompany cancer and chemotherapy.

SUPPORTING RESEARCH

Cannabis works in different ways to ease symptoms for most conditions a senior may have, from anxiety to psoriasis. For both healthy individuals and those in palliative care, CBD has been shown to be especially effective in lowering stress-related anxiety, most likely by working in conjunction with ECS (endocannabinoid system) receptors in the brain to reduce emotional memories linked to stressful situations. A report on the use of cannabis for oncology and palliative care, published in 2019 in the journal *Cancers*, chronicles the available evidence for treating pain, spasms, seizures, sleep disorders, nausea, vomiting, Tourette syndrome, and neuropathic pain with cannabis. This report also points up cannabis's relatively benign adverse effects, including no depressive effect on the respiratory system, making it a strong candidate for palliative care. THC, which has been found to be the stronger medicine for pain relief, can deliver a sense of well-being—even euphoria—to hospice patients and help ease them through their final days.

> "*My wife was in an extraordinary amount of pain. Her body was frail after going through round after round of chemotherapy and radiation therapy. She was hooked on morphine, had no appetite, couldn't eat, and was nauseous. It was 75 days after the bone marrow transplant, and it still didn't work. There was no hope left. She suffered with pain and anxiety. Initially we tracked down a dealer and tried cannabis at home. It worked and calmed her immediately. We got a cannabis card and were quickly able to adjust her dosage to get excellent control of her symptoms. We were very scared, but her death experience helped me start a wider conversation about treatments for cancer and help for others. So I guess it has all been for a very good reason.*"

> **—Jay, 41, Surgical Assistant**

Integrative Tip >>>>>

Chemotherapy-associated nerve damage and inactivity during treatment for cancer can drastically increase the risk of falls in cancer patients. Maintain your balance and protect yourself from falls by standing on one foot while you're getting dressed in the morning or when you're preparing your meals. If you lose your balance, the tabletop or kitchen counter will be right there to prevent you from falling.

12) Epilepsy and Seizures

Earlier, we chronicled the extraordinary story of Charlotte Figi. At the age of three, this little girl could not go through a day without a series of seizures—as many as 300 episodes a week. After hundreds of doctor visits, hospitalizations, and medications, her exhausted and terrified family finally sought help from cannabis, in the form of CBD, to control her symptoms. And it worked. Charlotte's condition, Dravet syndrome, is a rare form of epilepsy, a chronic neurological disorder.

According to the Epilepsy Foundation, 65 million people worldwide—and 3.4 million in the United States alone—have epilepsy. Here's what doctors know about this all-too common neurological disorder: Abnormal, overwhelming electrical signals, called "storms," originate in one section of the brain or perhaps sweep across it, triggering a seizure. Most often epilepsy begins in childhood, as a result of genetic connection. It may also be prompted by a mother's drug or alcohol use during pregnancy, or by an early infection or brain injury.

It may strike, too, with age, triggered by a stroke or a tumor in the brain, or even by Alzheimer's disease. According to researchers at Mayo Clinic, at least two "unprovoked seizures" are required for a person to be diagnosed with epilepsy. Having a single seizure, just one in a lifetime, perhaps as the result of extreme fever, trauma, drug abuse, or another extraordinarily stressful event, does not mean you have epilepsy.

Atonic, or absence, seizures occur when a person simply loses awareness and is basically absent. These seizures are usually brief, lasting only a few seconds. More often a seizure is tonic-clonic, or convulsive. In these cases, a person will fall down, experiencing repeated muscle contractions and jaw clenching, which, in rare cases, includes tongue injury. Following a seizure, a postictal phase—an altered state of consciousness—may last from five minutes to an hour as a person rests and recovers. During that time, one might experience drowsiness, nausea, and other disorienting symptoms. Unfortunately, there is no way to predict when the next seizure will strike. For one-third of seizure sufferers, the condition is drug-resistant; despite taking medications, breakthrough seizures still persist, leading to injury and inconvenience, such as not being able to drive. Needless to say, under those conditions, a person becomes housebound, and socialization suffers. Caregivers suffer from lack of contact, too.

Sometimes other conditions prompt epileptic symptoms. One of them is Dravet syndrome, a rare muscle disorder linked to gene mutation, which affects 1 out of 21,000 children in the United States. Epilepsy is frequently associated with Dravet syndrome. Another condition is Sturge-Weber syndrome, recognizable by port-wine stains on the face. Patients have glaucoma and vision problems, and 75 percent also have a significant seizure disorder. A third condition, Lennox-Gastaut syndrome, comes on in infancy and manifests as an atonic seizure, when muscles suddenly go limp, or an absence seizure, which causes brief lapses in awareness, sometimes accompanied by staring. While these various syndromes may impair development and remain lifelong conditions, ongoing research for medications and therapies are bringing hopeful breakthroughs.

The good news is that for most people with epilepsy, treatment with medication or surgery, in some cases, can control seizures. In the best outcomes, symptoms naturally subside, and some children may outgrow the condition altogether.

Current Remedies

Many antiseizure or antiepileptic medications on the market have treated epilepsy with varying degrees of success, but they come with unwanted side effects, such as fatigue, headache, nausea, tremors, weight gain, bone density loss, and speech and memory problems. Other therapies—for example, stimulating the vagus nerve, which passes through the neck—can help control seizures by sending electrical pulses to the brain.

According to Mayo Clinic, vagus nerve stimulation may help reduce seizures by up to 40 percent. Finally, in some cases, the portion of the brain that triggers seizures can be removed surgically.

For Dravet and Lennox-Gastaut syndromes, a combination of medicines to treat seizures may be recommended, along with diet therapy and brain stimulation. As of 2018, the FDA has approved two breakthrough drugs: Stiripentol for Dravet seizures, and Epidiolex® (cannabidiol, CBD) oral solution, which can be prescribed for both. (For more information about Epidiolex, see below.)

Why CBD or Medical Cannabis
Might Be the Answer

In June 2018, the US Food and Drug Administration approved Epidiolex in an oral solution to treat seizures in Lennox-Gastaut and Dravet syndromes, two severe forms of epilepsy. It is the first cannabis-based, FDA-approved drug for children two years of age and older who suffer from Dravet syndrome.

The use of cannabis to treat epilepsy has been recorded since the 10th century, but an FDA-approved medicine to treat the condition was not brought to market until 2009. The catalyst for this development was Charlotte Figi, the three-year-old who had suffered continuous seizures, some of which brought her close to death, since her first year of life. In 2009 Charlotte's desperate parents moved to Colorado to work with cannabis growers and researchers who recognized the profoundly calming effects of low-THC, high-CBD cannabis. They created a serum that soon reduced Charlotte's seizures from 50 events per day to 2 to 3 per month. After 20 months, Charlotte was weaned from antiepileptic drugs, thanks to the consistent performance of CBD. CNN's medical expert and correspondent Dr. Sanjay Gupta brought her story to millions of viewers across America, and soon the strain of cannabis that served Charlotte so well became known as Charlotte's Web. Epidiolex was subsequently produced in the United Kingdom for use in seizure disorders. According to a study reported in a 2017 issue of the journal *Epilepsy Currents*, 43 percent of patients who were administered the cannabidiol solution had at least a 50 percent reduction in the frequency of seizures—and studies continue. Epidiolex is the first and only prescription cannabidiol (CBD) for patients with epilepsy.

Almost all cannabis research for epilepsy has been done with CBD, rather than other cannabinoids—and that's exciting because CBD is readily available and legal in all 50 of the United States. In addition, surveys from five countries—the United States, Canada, Mexico, Israel, and Australia—are recording the benefits of CBD treatments, especially in children. The other good news is that caregivers are also experiencing benefits from the relief CBD brings to young patients.

Six randomized trials (where participants are randomly assigned to an experimental group) involving 555 pediatric, adolescent, and young adults who have seizure disorders are currently underway. Five of those trials are "gold standard trials," meaning they are double-blind (neither the participants nor the experimenters know who is receiving a particular treatment), placebo-controlled (an inactive substance, a placebo, is given to one group of participants, while the treatment being tested, usually a drug or vaccine, is given to another), *and* randomized. These trials are strong indicators that the data on CBD's effectiveness to manage seizures is compelling. At the onset of one 14-week study of Dravet syndrome patients, the average number of seizures per child was 12.4 per month. By the end of the study, there was a 50 percent reduction in seizures across the group—and 5 percent of the children became seizure-free. At the end of a 14-week study of 244 Lennox-Gastaut patients, there was a 41.9 percent decrease in seizure frequency among the children. Before starting CBD, they had averaged 80 seizures per month.

Some researchers think CBD works by changing the drug levels of antiseizure medication that the patient is already taking by impacting the breakdown of the medications in the liver. But most researchers now agree that CBD has a direct effect on seizures through the stimulation of CB receptors in the brain.

SUPPORTING RESEARCH

In early studies, researchers induced seizures in lab animals, then administered CBD. Afterward, the subjects not only had fewer seizures but also saw improvement in memory and repetitive-learning skills as well.

The lack of endocannabinoid tone (i.e., the overall state of your endocannabinoid system [ECS])* appears to play a role in launching seizures. In a 2017 study reported in the journal *Epilepsy Currents*, mice with uncontrolled seizures were shown to produce too little of the endocannabinoid anandamide to activate CB1 receptors in the brain. In the case of seizure control, the presence of adequate amounts of cannabinoids may be crucial. According to other ongoing trials, CBD can step in to help decrease the frequency of seizures and control the condition, most likely by interacting with both CB1 and CB2 receptors to keep information flowing smoothly in the brain. Disruption of the communication between neurons appears to trigger a seizure. CBD may also protect parts of the brain where seizures start. Researchers see promise for Epidiolex and other new, cannabis-based medicines currently being formulated. Edward Maa, MD, associate professor of neurology and chief of the Comprehensive Epilepsy Program at Denver Health Medial Center, Colorado, is currently leading trials to determine the role genetics play in the effect of cannabis on epilepsy patients. It's the first step, he says, "toward building a body of research on how and why medical marijuana can be used to treat epilepsy."

A quick reminder: The ECS, the endocannabinoid system, is a molecular system that regulates and balances many processes in the body, including immune response, communication between cells, appetite and metabolism, memory, and much more.

NOTE FROM DR. MARY

Despite significant findings that point toward the efficacy of CBD to help treat epilepsy, always work closely with a medical professional to dose CBD for this and any other condition, and do not stop any prescribed seizure medication. While the American Academy of Pediatrics notes that medical cannabinoids may be considered useful in the treatment of children and adolescents with debilitating diseases, there can also be adverse side effects, such as diarrhea and constipation. In addition to working closely with medical professionals, before administering cannabinoids as a medical treatment to a minor, always consult with legal counsel and make sure you have access to a poison control center. It is critical to the health of your child and for your own legal protection that you do not administer cannabinoid formulations, including CBD, to a child or a young adult without the approval of several professionals in your community. CBD is safe and legal in all 50 states. Administration to youths is the only time when people have run into legal trouble using CBD. Poison control is a toll-free number most parents will already have on hand in case of accidental ingestions.

A Thought on Strains and Products

When choosing CBD products, you can select products that are more or less processed. Full- or broad-spectrum CBD products are unprocessed extractions from the hemp plant and include all the cannabinoids, phytonutrients, and other potentially nourishing chemicals in the hemp plant. Using an unprocessed extraction like this may contribute to the entourage effect, where several different compounds in the formulation may work better together to provide the benefits of the hemp plant. Many people think the entourage effect is a very important part of managing conditions with CBD, and in some cases, full-spectrum botanicals may be more valuable. Alternatively, people can choose a CBD isolate—CBD that has undergone further distillation so that it is pure CBD without any other plant compounds.

Available studies show that it makes no difference whether you take a full-spectrum CBD product or an isolate product to help manage seizures. In managing seizures, both products appear to be equally beneficial.

> **"**My seizure disorder led to small seizures, also known as petit mal seizures, which sometimes went unnoticed by other people. In times of stress, I could have many small seizures every day and then sometimes go for a week without any. I would never use marijuana for recreational purposes. For me, it is a medicine and not a drug in the negative sense of the word. I use marijuana as another way to help myself have a more normal life. **"**

—Eleesha, 36, Retail Sales Associate

Integrative Tip >>>>>

Use a lot of seasonings in your food. Many spices and herbs are highly concentrated sources of precious terpenes and antioxidants that can help balance and tone the ECS, especially when ingested in combination with cannabis. Terpenes, compounds found in foods and in cannabis, stimulate the ECS without using CBD or other cannabinoids. Look to fresh lemon for limonene (a terpene) and to basil and black pepper for pinene (also a terpene). These foods are antioxidants, too.

13) Eye Health

The ancient Babylonians believed that demons caused eye problems; if you squinted at someone, you were accused of giving them the evil eye. A good eye-rubbing with an onion might've be in store for you. Times have changed, and while we wear eyeglasses and contact lenses and go through corrective surgery to escape evil-eye syndrome, we still can take measures to protect and maintain the precious gift of sight—the ability to experience this living world in three dimensions.

Some eye diseases are genetic, and others are unstoppable as we age and experience the regular wear and tear of life. The numbers are sobering:

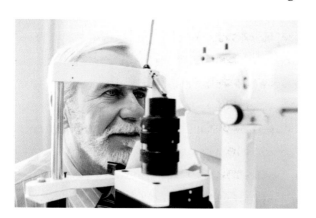

By 2030 nearly 60 million Americans will suffer from sight loss or blindness, including glaucoma, cataracts, macular degeneration, and retinopathy. According to the American Academy of Ophthalmology, glaucoma is among the greatest threats, with 7.2 million Americans projected to experience the disease in 2050. Glaucoma is a complex disease, where the flow of fluid inside the eye slows down, causing pressure to build and gradually damaging the optic nerve and destroying sight.

Fortunately, a cataract, a film that grows over the lens as we age, or if the eye has been injured, can be removed through a time-tested standard procedure with a brief recovery period. Retinopathy is a complication of diabetes in which vessels in the retina—the light-sensitive tissue at the back of the eye—may swell or grow abnormally. Macular degeneration destroys the macula, the part of the eye located in the retina that allows us to see objects clearly; chances for development of this condition skyrocket after the age of 80. Ongoing ophthalmological advances in measuring changes in the structure and contents of the eye are bringing everyone a little closer to those clear skies in which one can see forever.

Current Remedies

Good practices can help keep your eyes healthy and your sight clear for decades: Shield them from bright sun; if you wear eye makeup, clean it off thoroughly each night; keep blood vessels healthy and circulation in tip-top shape by exercising every day and eating a diet filled with vitamins and omega-3-rich fish, nuts, fruits, and vegetables. The brighter the fruit and veggie colors (red peppers, orange carrots, deep-green spinach), the more packed they are with eye-protective vitamins A, C, and E.

Serious eye diseases are not the only conditions to be aware of: Your eyes can become inflamed through allergies, conjunctivitis (aka pink eye), or an eyelid inflammation due to a bacterial infection or perhaps a blocked gland near the eyelashes. If you have symptoms of any of those conditions, first of all, don't rub your eyes, and second, see a doctor. They may prescribe antibiotics for bacterial infection or steroid eye drops to control inflammation. An over-the-counter artificial-tears product will keep your eyes lubricated. Always keep the affected area as pristine as possible, and apply a clean, warm compress to remove crust that may build up overnight.

Why CBD or Medical Cannabis Might Be the Answer

Cannabis, studies show, is good for the eyes. It reduces inflammation and blocks harmful oxidation. It also causes blood vessels to dilate, sending extra healing blood flow to the eyes. THC is the cannabinoid most closely associated with blood vessel dilation. While it makes for healthy eyes, it also turns eyes red and bloodshot. Stay hydrated and also consider using lubricating eye drops if your eyes get uncomfortably dry. To avoid red, bloodshot eyes linked to THC, the simplest solution is to reduce the amount of THC in the product you're using. CBD and THC both have neuroprotective properties; that is, they help protect cells from damage and guard those cells that have already been damaged from devolving into chronic disease. Studies have shown that CBD and THC can help reduce small rips in the retina that trigger macular degeneration. THC has also been shown to reduce the pressure buildup that causes glaucoma. Some patients taking oral forms of cannabis have reported eye improvement for near- or farsightedness.

SUPPORTING RESEARCH

A 2016 study published in the journal *Neural Plasticity* explains that the retina is actually part of the central nervous system (CNS), connected to the CNS by the optic nerve. Therefore the endocannabinoid system (ECS) receptors CB1 and CB2 that are so richly distributed throughout the CNS are also in the retina. They play a major role in the retina's biological makeup, protection, and function, including the efficient processing of light, which helps us to see. Researchers hold that the use of cannabis not only has the potential to boost light processing and other retinal function; it is also likely that synthetic cannabinoid products will play a role in preventing and treating retinal disease in the future. In addition, a National Institutes of Health (NIH)–supported study in a 2018 issue of the journal

Cannabis and Cannabinoid Research underscores that CBD, along with THC, interacts with CB1 and CB2 receptors to reduce the pain and inflammation from surface eye injury that leads to cataracts. While early testing showed that cannabis can relieve the ocular pressure of glaucoma, as of 2020, the NIH and the American Academy of Ophthalmology strongly advise against its use for treating glaucoma, saying that more testing is needed to determine its effectiveness.

> **❝***I was diagnosed with glaucoma and soon found that nothing worked on my glaucoma except cannabis. I believed all the lies, [about using marijuana] and now I believe that ignorance blinds us. I'm lucky because I don't have to take pills and other pills to deal with the side effects of the first pill. Marijuana is the only medication I need.*❞
>
> —**Sally, 72, Retired**

Integrative Tip > > > > >
Drink high-antioxidant hibiscus tea all day long. Hibiscus tea has ten times the antioxidants of green tea and tastes like fruit punch, especially with a squeeze of lemon.

14) Headache

Headache. It's the most common reason people miss school or work—and the fourth most common reason for a visit to the emergency room.

Mayo Clinic defines *headache* as "pain in any region of the head"—on one or both sides, focused in one location, or starting at one point and radiating across the head, sometimes with a viselike grip. Headache pain can be sharp, throbbing, or dull. And a headache can last for less than an hour or up to days.

If variety is the spice of life, headaches are the extra-hot vindaloo. The International Headache Society classifies 150 kinds of headaches as either primary or secondary. Primary headaches include the common *tension headache*, often the result of stress, aggravated by dehydration, poor posture, and lack of sleep; *cluster headaches*, which occur in cyclical patterns or "cluster" around one eye; and *migraine*, the most severe kind of headache, often begins with (or is accompanied by) an aura, which can include visual disturbances, such as flashing lights or blind spots. Migraine can cause nausea, vomiting, and extreme sensitivity to light and sound, requiring the sufferer to retreat to dark, quiet quarters, sometimes for as long as 72 hours. If you experience migraines, you are not alone: One billion people around the world, including 39 million in the United States alone, suffer from these severe headaches. Although primary headaches can be genetically linked, most are prompted by chemical activity in your brain, the nerves and blood vessels surrounding your skull, or the muscles in your head and neck.

Secondary headaches are triggered by other conditions—such as fever, infection, high blood pressure, brain tumor, overmedication, and psychiatric and nerve disorders—and can aggravate the pain-sensitive nerves of the head. These headaches can be extremely serious, indicating meningitis, encephalitis, or stroke. Call 911 immediately if you are experiencing an unusually sudden or severe headache, accompanied by confusion, fainting, or an extreme fever over 101°F.

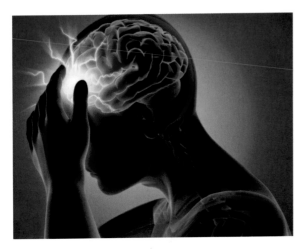

According to a 2018 issue of *Headache: The Journal of Head and Face Pain*, a study of adults across the United States showed that migraine and severe headaches affect one out of every six Americans. Rates of headache over a three-month period were found to be highest in women, especially those of reproductive age, and in American Indian communities. The unemployed, the elderly, and those with disabilities were also shown to be at risk. A common thread connecting all these groups? Stress, say experts. (To discover more about that trigger condition, see page 136.)

Current Treatments

Tension headaches—and some migraines—may resolve with over-the-counter remedies like ibuprofen and acetaminophen. Other, stronger medications are prescribed for most migraines and for cluster headaches. Triptans, for instance, may be prescribed for migraine because they block pain pathways to the brain. When other medications don't work, opioids may be prescribed; however, because of their strength and addictive quality the American Headache Society does not recommend them. All pharmaceuticals may have side effects, especially for women who are pregnant or breastfeeding. For that reason, a 2017 issue of the journal *Medical Clinics of North America* reports that 82 percent of people with migraines seek alternative options. The American Academy of Neurology cites adequate sleep and hydration, acupuncture, and dietary supplements such as magnesium and vitamin B_2 as potential migraine preventers. Because stress is considered the primary trigger for migraine, relaxation therapy is key: Massage, yoga, meditation, or a relaxing soak could help.

Why CBD or Medical Cannabis Might Be the Answer

A harbinger of hope for headache sufferers, a 2017 issue of the journal *Cannabis and Cannabinoid Research* reported that "CBD has shown efficacy for headache-related conditions." Cannabinoids could likely stimulate the ECS (endocannabinoid system) and help treat the pain at its source, and human clinical trials are the next step in potentially making cannabinoids a mainstream headache medication. Just two years later, in 2019, a groundbreaking study in the journal *Pain* reported that inhaled cannabis can reduce self-reported headache severity by 47.3 percent and migraine severity by 49.6 percent. While previous studies were based on patients' past experiences, the *Pain* study collected and analyzed big data from patients using cannabis in real time.

Only one other clinical trial, contending that cannabis was better than ibuprofen for headache relief, has been carried out, but it focused on a synthetic cannabinoid drug called nabilone. In the *Pain* study, researchers found that cannabis, unlike pharmaceuticals, did not trigger "overuse headache" (a pattern of increased headaches caused by taking too much headache medication). However, patients did use larger doses over time and possibly developed a tolerance to it.

SUPPORTING RESEARCH

Many stress-triggered headaches can be soothed by cannabis, which prompts the ECS to release soothing chemicals like serotonin and dopamine. Migraines are a different story. Pain research shows that these severe headaches may occur because of what neurologist and cannabis educator Ethan Russo terms "endocannabinoid deficiency syndrome." The intense pain of the headache also has to do with an unusual response to inflammation. A migraine may be triggered by bright lights, chemicals, premenstrual hormones, unpleasant smells, allergies, anxiety, or chronic pain disorders. In a healthy ECS, triggers like those cause the release of endocannabinoids to balance the system and keep pain in check. But for people who suffer from migraines, that release doesn't seem to happen. Instead, other chemicals flood the system, dilating blood vessels on the surface of the brain, increasing pressure and inflammation, and prompting pain.

As far back as 2008, in an issue of the journal *Neuroendocrinology Letters*, Dr. Russo explained that cannabinoids have been shown to "block spinal, peripheral, and gastrointestinal mechanisms that promote pain in headache, fibromyalgia, IBS, and related disorders." A 2010 study in another research journal, *Experimental Neurology*, supported Dr. Russo's work and commented that activating the ECS with cannabinoids may be "a promising therapeutic tool" for fighting inflammation and migraine pain. The 2019 study in the journal *Pain*, noted previously, is a major step in that direction. But there are still a number of fine points, yet to be determined, as to how cannabis can alleviate migraine. Researchers have found that while cannabis concentrates, such as oils, help lower headache severity more than the cannabis flower used in smoking, there is no difference in relief between THC-rich or CBD-rich products. That may mean that other cannabis components, such as terpenes, can relieve more pain than the better-known and more heavily researched cannabinoids.

"I sustained a terrible concussion playing sports, and the post-concussive headache syndrome has persisted. Riding in a car was an awful experience. Over the years I have been prescribed 20 different medications to deal with the pain. I was eventually on Ativan three times a day, antidepressants, and opioid painkillers, leaving me with brain fog and depleting me of my personality. I started to look into alternative healers, and this research led me to chiropractors and an acupuncturist and also to cannabis. After comparing studies, I used cannabis and had unbelievable, nearly instantaneous headache pain relief. Now I am able to laugh and enjoy life with my friends and family, and I'm back to working full time."

—Kristine, 28, Legal Assistant

Integrative Tip > > > > >

Get outdoors. The fresh air is good for you, and grounding also helps release harmful electrical charges that accumulate over the day and may impact your immunity and brain function. Weather permitting, go outdoors and take off your shoes and socks. Let your bare feet connect with the earth; this is known as "grounding."

15) Heart Health/Heart Disease

The heart is the center of our being. First analyzed 2,500 years ago by the legendary healer Hippocrates, the heart and the life-giving properties of this vital organ are still analyzed with awe. For us to live, our heart must function. Tragically, a "broken heart" is the leading cause of death in the United States. Each year one in four people will die of heart disease—that's more than 600,000 Americans.

Why does heart function go awry? Cardiovascular disease—*cardio* means "heart" and *vascular* means "vein"—is the number one cause. Basically, poor diet, lack of exercise, smoking, stress, a disease like diabetes, or genetics prompt the body to overproduce a kind of fatty plaque. This plaque piles up on artery walls, stiffening them and creating a blockage that compromises blood flow, keeping it from reaching and nourishing tissues and organs—including your heart. Consequently, the body becomes inflamed. As blockage increases, the heart works overtime to pump blood to other parts of the body. Blood pressure—the force that pushes blood through the veins—rises, causing hypertension followed by heart attack or stroke.

Plaque contains a waxy, fatty ingredient called cholesterol. While cholesterol is vital for lining cells and helping the body synthesize hormones and vitamin D, among other life-giving functions, too much can combine with other substances in the blood to form vein-narrowing plaque. The result is heart attack—an abrupt discontinuation of blood flow to the heart. For patients who are experiencing a heart attack, the development of abnormal dangerous heart rhythms is a serious complication that can further compromise the patient and contribute to prolonged hospitalization and increased risk of death.

Other heart conditions, such as congestive heart failure, valve malfunction, thickening of the heart walls, or arrhythmia (an irregular heartbeat) may be genetic, caused by a virus, or the side effect of a toxin or drug. Researchers work overtime to determine how these conditions can be addressed so that every awe-inspiring heart can keep giving its owner a long and wondrous life.

Current Treatments

An ounce of prevention is worth a pound of cure. For your heart, an ounce of prevention is absolutely mandatory. To avoid heart disease, you need to engage in moderate exercise; adopt a low-stress and smoke-free lifestyle; follow a low-salt diet rich in fruits, vegetables, and foods containing omega-3 fatty acids—almonds and salmon are examples; and limit alcohol intake. All these practices have anti-inflammatory effects that can help control unwanted cholesterol and venous plaque buildup.

Some kinds of heart disease must be treated with medications. Statins, like atorvastatin, better known as Lipitor®, may be prescribed to keep cholesterol in check. For heart failure or arrhythmia, a beta blocker, such as carvedilol (sold under the brand name Coreg®, among others), may be needed to keep heart rate regular, reduce blood pressure, and limit or even reverse existing heart damage. If heart surgery is required, a blood thinner, such as warfarin (Coumadin®), may be prescribed to avoid life-threatening blood clots.

Why CBD or Medical Cannabis Might Be the Answer

The American Heart Association believes that cannabis contributes to the development of heart disease and heart attacks. The literature is rife with case reports of people of all ages who used cannabinoid formulations prior to a heart attack; people who present with acute coronary syndrome after consumption of cannabinoid formulations; or young people with normal coronary arteries who experienced a heart attack after physical exertion—also related to use of cannabinoid formulations and CBD. From those case reports, it would seem that if consumption of cannabis is anywhere in a victim's recent past, the only cause for the heart condition would be cannabis.

However, when you actually look at the literature, it becomes clear that the case reports that receive the most attention from research publications sensationalize and support the existing bias. Within cannabis research and reporting, there is considerable bias toward the negative effects of cannabis. With the advent of electronic medical records, however, it is becoming easier to determine if there is an actual correlation between the use of cannabis and heart disease.

Longitudinal studies (research conducted over a period of time, sometimes many years, observing the same subjects) have revealed that cannabis likely does *not* have a significant impact on long-term mortality. There may be a short-term effect at the time of administration that results in heart-rate elevation or modest changes in blood pressure—and I certainly have patients who describe these responses when they're consuming cannabis—but it does not appear to increase the risk of heart attack or death in either the short or the long term.

Overall, the beneficial effects of cannabinoid formulations on the cardiovascular system far outweigh the risks. By helping to control common risk factors for heart disease—such as reducing cigarette smoking; decreasing the rate of obesity and diabetes and lowering fasting insulin levels, prompting smaller waist circumference; and improving HDL/LDL cholesterol ratios and triglyceride levels—cannabis provides protection against heart disease and heart attack.

The other interesting and novel way cannabis may protect the heart is by keeping it from developing dangerous irregular heart rhythms that can exacerbate heart failure or heart attack and prolong a patient's hospitalization or increase the risk of death. Researchers have found that people using cannabinoid formulations are less likely to experience atrial fibrillation (a common irregular heart rhythm) as a complication of heart failure. In fact, in the first-ever human study presented at the 2018 Heart Rhythm Society Scientific Sessions in San Diego, it was shown that atrial fibrillation, as a consequence of heart failure, was less likely to develop in people using cannabis prior to their admission to the hospital.

SUPPORTING RESEARCH

In one study, researchers concluded that CBD can help blood vessels relax and increase in diameter, so that blood flow to the heart remains consistent, flowing around plaque buildup in the vessel and, importantly, helping to prevent myocardial infarction (heart attack) and stroke. Over years of research, CBD has also been found to reduce inflammation and oxidation in all organs, including the heart. A 2013 study in the *British Journal of Pharmacology* not only supported its role in relaxing arterial walls and increasing blood flow, it also noted that CBD helped stem plaque formation and protected arteries against damage from inflammation. Those improvements—better blood flow, less plaque buildup, reduced inflammation, and the like—help lower blood pressure and counteract hypertension, which leads to heart disease. Another study, published in *American Journal of Cardiology* in 2016, with more than 4,500 participants showed that cannabis users had higher levels of good cholesterol (HDL). Research published in the 2015 journal *Obesity*, which analyzed 700 Inuit cannabis users, showed both a rise in HDL and a drop in levels of bad cholesterol (LDL). CBD is also a well-known antioxidant, which protects healthy cells from damage. Scientists see a potential role for CBD in protecting the heart from cardiomyopathy, a disease that is sometimes triggered by diabetes in which the heart muscle becomes so rigid that it can't pump blood efficiently to the rest of the body. Finally, hemp seed oil, which can easily be purchased at a health food store, is packed with heart-protective omega-3s.

❝My lifetime battle with crippling anxiety is over. Almost better yet, the weight gain I experienced from antidepressants has slowly resolved, and I'm back to my high school weight. The high cholesterol and prediabetes that I was dealing with when I was overweight have completely resolved. I have a strong family history of heart disease, and I feel safer and healthier now that these metabolic conditions have reversed.❞

—Pat, 47, Psychologist

Integrative Tip >>>>>
Through his lifetime of travel and study around the world, researcher Dan Buettner identified Blue Zones, places where heart-healthy, long-lived populations are concentrated in regions where diets are rich in fruits, vegetables, and fish; people work outdoors well into their eighties and after; smoking is rare; and lifestyle practices and spiritual outlook keep stress at bay. When preparing heart-healthy meat-and-vegetable combos, you can almost always double the vegetables and cut the meat in half to increase the nutritional density of the meal and reduce calorie counts while still feeling full.

16) Immune System Health

Have you ever thought of how complex and miraculous the immune system function must be to allow a completely foreign object like a baby to thrive and grow inside a woman for nine months?

Whether that "foreign object" is a cause for joy or worry, your immune system is on the case, determining if it should be left in place or ousted. It's amazing that the immune system can see something as foreign as an entirely different human being inside a pregnant woman and leave it alone—and then aggressively fight other aliens like strep and staph infections in the upper respiratory system or on the skin. On the other hand, it's astonishing that the immune system can also go completely awry and attack a perfectly healthy thyroid or pancreas, leading to unwanted hypothyroidism or diabetes or 180 other conditions that have been associated with autoimmune phenomena—that is, when the immune system mistakenly attacks healthy body tissue.

When operating smoothly, the immune system is highly selective. In the case of a foreign bacterium like strep, cells in the body called antigen-presenting cells show a portion of the antigen, in this case the harmful bacteria, to the immune system. The immune system, in turn, gives it a thumbs-up (baby) or a thumbs-down (strep). If the immune system recognizes the bacterium from a previous encounter, it can react even faster. Next, the immune system sends out antibodies to kill the bacteria. It also creates commander molecules called cytokines. Cytokines prompt production of more antibodies and also direct the antibodies to fight bacteria. At the same time, however, cytokines trigger fever, body aches, inflammation, and nausea. If too many are produced, symptoms are overly severe and can lead to complications. The good news is that an efficient immune system can wipe out bad bacteria in a few days and stop cytokine production. Side effects will dissipate.

The actions of the immune response described above are normal, but when the immune response goes awry, there is also an autoimmune response. This happens because vast parts of the immune system are designed to manage chronic infections, perhaps from parasites or tuberculosis. With medical advancements such as vaccines, the immune system has had a lot of outside help, and those conditions have been eradicated for the most part. Now the immune system needs to look elsewhere to do its work and sometimes runs amok, searching for trouble around the body. It may seek out inflammatory situations resulting from a poor diet and lifestyle that prompt conditions such as asthma and allergies. It may also go after the pancreas or thyroid in an attempt to protect the body from what it mistakenly perceives as a foreign object. With 180 different autoimmune diseases out there, we need to determine how to get the immune system to respond appropriately. Keeping it strong and directed may depend both on reining in inflammatory lifestyles and suppressing the immune system to keep it from attacking other body systems.

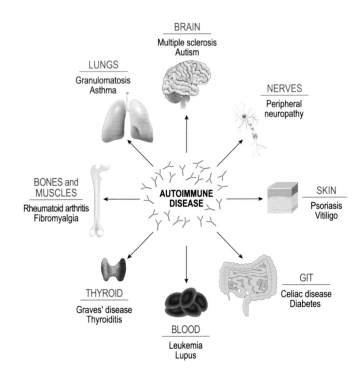

Current Remedies

According to Mayo Clinic, the immune system can be enhanced by therapies such as immunoglobulin, which boosts antibodies to fight infection; interferon-gamma therapy, which stimulates immune system cells; and cell-growth therapy, which increases immune-boosting white blood cells. In addition, stem-cell transplants can address extremely deficient immune systems. Fortunately, a host of simple lifestyle choices and a few nutritional supplements can arm your immune system and make it much more resilient. First and foremost: Take care of yourself. Cut back on stressful living. Sleep eight hours a night. Ditch processed foods that are loaded with inflammatory sugars and fats. Spend time with friends and loved ones. Exercise. When you're food shopping, remember: Plants are top immune boosters, both antioxidant and anti-inflammatory. Buy mushrooms for their polysaccharides—beta-glucans, which are exceptional immune enhancers. Add to your diet fish that contain immune-supporting vitamin D and inflammation-fighting omega-3 fatty acids, plus zinc-rich nuts and fermented probiotics.

Why CBD or Medical Cannabis Might Be the Answer

Could CBD and other cannabinoids help modulate your immune response, both to colds and flu, as well as to more complicated autoimmune conditions like thyroid disease? The answer appears to be yes. A 2015 study of 168 patients showed that lifetime cannabinoid users had lower levels of a highly inflammatory protein called tumor necrosis factor (TNF), often overproduced in rheumatoid arthritis patients. Cannabinoids were also found to reduce the production of potentially inflammatory cytokines (proteins released by the immune system). A 2014 Egyptian study published in *Inflammopharmacology* revealed that cannabinoid users had a balanced production of cytokines, allowing their bodies to better respond to infection.

In a 2013 study on cannabis use reported in the journal *Inflammatory Bowel Diseases*, 292 patients with the autoimmune condition irritable bowel disease saw an average 16 percent reduction in symptoms of abdominal pain, nausea, and diarrhea and reduced inflammation in measurable ways on multiple different cytokines.

In autoimmune diseases that affect the central nervous system, such as MS and ALS, cannabinoids may not only help calm spasms, they may also control the progression of the disease as it unfolds in the body.

SUPPORTING RESEARCH

There is a close relationship between cannabinoids and the immune system. CB2 receptors are richly present throughout the body's immune system, especially on the spleen and lymph nodes, helping control our immune responses and regulate the amount of cytokines produced. Research in both human and mouse models show that pretreating with CBD before exposure to flu can reduce the overdevelopment of cytokines by as much as 87 percent. While cytokines are doing their work telling the immune cells to fight bacteria, there are now fewer of them also triggering nausea, body aches, and potential life-threatening complications. This gives a patient a simpler course through cold or flu.

In the case of an autoimmune condition, we know that CB receptors and endocannabinoids are already reacting strongly to immune responses and inflammatory responses. For instance, patients with rheumatoid arthritis (RA) have elevated CB receptors in their knees and elevated amounts of the endocannabinoids anandamide and 2-AG in the synovial fluid of the affected joints. This means the ECS (endocannabinoid system) is already trying to reduce the inflammation from the RA.

Cannabinoids are powerful anti-inflammatory molecules that, unlike many antibiotics, appear to readily cross the blood-brain barrier and have a significant impact on reducing the chronic inflammation that promotes autoimmune diseases in the central nervous system, such as MS and ALS. For patients with those diseases, cannabinoids can help control both spasms and pain.

" *Celiac disease left me with persistent fatigue, pain, random ankle swelling, and hair loss. I added cannabis to my treatment regimen after reading about research in Israel that showed a significant reduction in symptoms for patients with Crohn's disease. I've been taking a tincture every eight hours, and that's made it possible for me to call in sick a lot less and also spend more time with my partner.* "

—Lewis, 25,
Elementary School Admissions Officer

Integrative Tip $>>>>>$

Don't forget that the tongue is a reservoir for bacteria that cause tooth decay and bad breath. Clean your tongue each day in addition to brushing, flossing, and regular dental visits for optimum dental health.

17) Inflammation

On page 21 we introduced inflammation as a root cause of ailments and conditions ranging from arthritis to cancer. In this section, we'll discuss how inflammation begins and the crucial role it plays not only in various ailments but in healing as well. For example, when you nick your finger with a knife while fixing dinner, your immune system sends an army of white blood cells to the area to fight infection. The ensuing battle turns the area pink and puffy and warm as your skin knits together, heals, and becomes smooth again. That action, called acute inflammation, is quick, direct, and contained. It also occurs with a sprain, a bruise, or an upper-respiratory infection. In all those cases, healing depends on care. By protecting and resting the area, you allow your system to function efficiently, address the injury, and get back to regular programming. In some cases, however, a wound doesn't heal right away and chronic inflammation results, as white blood cells continue their attack against infection. Catalysts for chronic inflammation can also be long-term stress, lack of sleep, depression, and anxiety. Each of those conditions is a continual assault on the body that can't

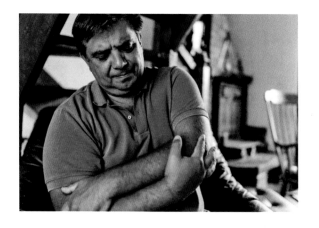

be healed by the action of normal white blood cells. Gradually the body experiences a breakdown due to oxidation, the same process that causes metal to rust. A chronically troubled body generates atoms called free radicals, which lack a full set of electrons. Consequently, those partial atoms begin to steal electrons from full atoms, resulting in a chain reaction that "rusts" your body. Aging speeds up, digestion is compromised, and joints become inflamed. But that's not all. Cell oxidation can give rise to diabetes, heart disease, cancer, and many other conditions.

Current Treatments

NSAIDs—nonsteroidal anti-inflammatory drugs—are perhaps the most common treatment for inflammation, and you'll likely know two of them well: over-the-counter ibuprofen (aka Advil) and naproxen (aka Aleve®). In particular, NSAIDs focus on reducing swelling, inflammation, and the accompanying pain in joints and muscles. These drugs also address fever and general aches and

pains. However, taking too much of them over a long period can break down tissue in the stomach and gastrointestinal tract and cause internal bleeding and more serious complications.

Why CBD or Medical Cannabis Might Be the Answer

For decades, research has pinpointed cannabis as a treatment for chronic inflammation. In the 2018 edition of the journal *Cannabis and Cannabinoid Research*, arthritis patients reported that cannabis worked "very well" or "moderately well" to relieve inflamed joints without the use of supplemental drugs like ibuprofen or prescription steroids such as prednisone. Another study in the *Canadian Medical Association Journal* indicated that arthritis patients reported decreased pain after being treated with cannabis. Animal data also show significant reductions in proinflammatory cytokine (which plays a central role in inflammatory diseases). Strong clinical studies archived in the National Institutes of Health (NIH) Library over a 30-year period demonstrate the anti-inflammatory effect of cannabis on chronic inflammation and the diseases it prompts, including heart disease, diabetes, inflammatory bowel disease, and many other conditions that we'll discuss in the following pages.

SUPPORTING RESEARCH

CBD and THC have been found to help stimulate the endocannabinoid receptors CB1 and CB2, which produce anti-inflammatory responses.

An article in a 2018 issue of the journal *Molecule* compiled preclinical and clinical data showing that certain endocannabinoids, which are produced by the ECS (endocannabinoid system), can have anti-inflammatory effects when targeting CB2 receptors. The data show that ingesting phytocannabinoid cannabis may reduce low-grade, chronic inflammation associated with neuropathic pain by targeting CB1 and CB2 receptors. Consequently, by helping to control inflammation through the ECS, cannabis may also help relieve the impact of inflammation on cell oxidation, which promotes other inflammatory conditions, from Alzheimer's to multiple sclerosis.

" *My inflammation is easy to spot and doesn't require complicated testing to uncover its presence. There's an area of chronic inflammation in the form of a rash on my left ankle, which is intermittently itchy and flaky. I also get deep pimples on my face that leave spots for months after I pop and put steroid cream on them. After several courses of treatment with a combination high-potency steroid and high-potency antifungal prescription therapy, my doctor recommended a topical cannabis formulation. That was a year ago, and I haven't seen the rash since. I also started using it after I pop my pimples, and they heal without the lingering spot.* "

—Martin, 51, Teacher

An anti-inflammatory diet is a frontline defense against the evils of inflammation. For patients with rheumatoid arthritis, the Arthritis Foundation suggests following a Mediterranean diet high in fish, vegetables, and olive oil, supplemented by whole grains, fruits, low-fat cheeses, and even a little red wine. A tomato salad with olives and chunks of cucumber and feta cheese, for example, is a tasty way to help lead the charge against inflammatory invaders.

18) Influenza

At some point, nearly everyone contracts influenza, better known as the flu. This highly contagious respiratory illness infects up to 20 percent of Americans every year. Near the end of the 2019–2020 season, the Centers for Disease Control and Prevention (CDC) estimated that there were 32 million cases of flu in the United States, with 310,000 people hospitalized. Some 18,000 of those cases resulted in death. Those most vulnerable to flu are individuals over 65 years of age, infants under 2 years old, pregnant women, and people with chronic illness. In addition, other viruses, such as parainfluenza and rhinovirus, present with similar symptoms at the same time of year, making flu difficult to diagnose without testing. Finally, the emergence of the novel coronavirus strain COVID-19 has led to worldwide quarantine.

If flu is so commonplace, how can it be so deadly? First of all, unlike viral infections such as chicken pox that stimulate lifelong immunity, flu viruses undergo continual genetic modification, with new challenges to our immune system each season. Second, any kind of flu virus is strong and tenacious—and it sneaks up on us. Not only does it spread easily from coughers and sneezers sitting next to you on the subway, students in your class, or coworkers at the office, but it hangs around on doorknobs, elevator buttons, faucets, cell phones, and countertops. If you buy your groceries at an electronic self-checkout that was just used by a coughing, sneezing shopper and then you inadvertently rub your eyes, you've just self-infected.

Within 14 days' time, a sore throat and stuffy nose set in. A cough develops. Headache, fever, chills, and body aches follow. Unlike the common cold, which settles in from the neck up, influenza causes full-body distress. The fever and aches are actually good—they're signs of a strong immune system fighting off an unwanted visitor. Cytokines—proteins that are released by the immune system to fight disease—trigger inflammation and thus fever and body ache. While these symptoms are uncomfortable, they're signs that your body is actively fighting the disease. (See "Immune System Health," page 93.)

Very important: *The day before* you exhibit flu symptoms, you are already contagious. So as soon as your throat starts feeling scratchy and you have a stuffy nose, stay home so as not to infect anyone else—and get better yourself. For most people, lying low and letting the flu run its course

are the best answers. With a healthy system, flu can resolve within three to four days; if your system is compromised, however, two weeks or more to rest and recover may be required, with more dire consequences. When quarantine is indicated, settle in at home with plenty of supplies to take good care of yourself. Wear a mask anytime you're in the community, and practice infection control by maintaining good hygiene. First and foremost, wash your hands!

In 2004 the CDC began testing subsets of genes that were responsible for a major influenza pandemic that broke out in 1918 at the end of World War I, killing 50 million people worldwide—more casualties than from the war itself. This 21st-century research led researchers to identify the virus's key genes and the ongoing development of antiviral drugs to fight similar viruses.

Current Treatments

While a yearly flu vaccination has long been recommended by the CDC for anyone over six months of age, mounting research systematically proves that flu shots are not 100 percent effective. Make sure to combine a healthy diet, excellent sleep, and regular exercise with your vaccinations to maximize their value for you. When flu season strikes, prevention by practicing good hygiene is the frontline defense. That means washing your hands often, covering your mouth and nose when you sneeze, and immediately disposing of used tissues. And if flu takes you down? Doctors usually recommend bed rest and plenty of fluids. A severe infection, however, may require an antiviral prescription, such as oseltamivir (Tamiflu®), which is oral; zanamivir (Relenza®), which is inhaled; or other similar medications to help relieve symptoms and shorten the bout.

Why CBD or Medical Cannabis Might Be the Answer

There have been a number of studies focusing on viral respiratory infections and how the body responds to them. Over the last two decades, some of those studies have focused on how CBD and other cannabinoids could potentially impact that response. Pretreating patients with CBD, for example, might help boost their immune system against infection in the first place, as well as help them not to feel *so* sick when they do get sick.

When flu epidemics hit your community, it's likely you'll get some kind of upper-respiratory infection, as often as four times a year. Managing how your body responds to those infections is a key part of staying productive, healthy, and happy during cold and flu season. If pretreating is found to be effective, you may be putting CBD next to Tamiflu in your medicine cabinet in the not-too-distant future.

SUPPORTING RESEARCH

Decades of studies, including research published in a 2017 edition of the journal *Frontiers in Immunology,* point to the interaction of the endocannabinoid system and cannabinoids with the immune system to regulate inflammation and other disease responses. (See "Immune System Health," page 93.)

Based on ongoing research, including a 2014 study in *Inflammopharmacology,* it turns out that cannabinoids like CBD can help suppress the production of cytokines in the body. While the immune system produces cytokines to help fight flu and other infection through helpful inflammation, the release of too many cytokines creates excessive inflammation, with accompanying body aches, nausea, headache, and other flu symptoms that make us feel terrible. In one study involving mice, subjects were either pretreated with CBD or had no treatment. When the mice that had been pretreated with CBD were exposed to the flu virus, their symptoms were reduced by up to 87 percent—probably due to the significant reduction of cytokines. These mice continued their usual activities, while their counterparts were sluggish.

The Egyptian study cited above and others like it shine a light on the potential use of CBD pretreatment to prepare us for flu season. To move this along, we could look at human models in a randomized trial, where some participants would be treated with CBD or other cannabinoids and some wouldn't. We could then analyze each person's response to flu and other infections. If the results are as promising as the mouse studies, we could be using CBD during flu season to help control the disease in our communities.

> "I always smoke cannabis when I have a cold. I have a medical cannabis card already for my back pain. Sometimes it makes me a little dizzy, especially if my ears are already plugged up. And I don't think it works well with NyQuil®. I feel like I get sick a lot, but if I take it when I have a sore throat, it overall eases my symptoms until I can recuperate."
>
> —Shawn, 32, Finance Professional

Integrative Tip >>>>>

Your grandmother was right! Drinking warm chicken soup when you have the flu does help—by soothing your sore throat and easing congestion. Soup or any other steaming liquid keeps your respiratory system hydrated and thins mucus so you can cough it up. By clearing out your lungs, you'll keep infection from setting in.

19) Insomnia

Do you have trouble sleeping? You're not alone. Nearly 50 percent of adults in the United States deal with insomnia on a regular basis. And make no mistake: Even occasional insomnia could be secretly doing more damage than leaving you tired or distracted. Lack of sleep affects growth and stress hormones, your immune system, appetite, breathing, blood pressure, and cardiovascular health. On the other hand, research shows that the benefits of sleep are countless. Did you know that your cells actually regenerate and repair while you sleep? And brain function improves because sleep enhances the communication of brain-based nerve cells and supports the bodily process of breaking down and removing toxins your brain has built up during your waking hours. In addition, sleep promotes healthy weight, lowered risk for serious health problems like diabetes and heart disease, reduced stress, and improved mood. And getting more sleep can create a massive transformation in your life. It is often the secret weapon to creating more energy, which allows you to perform at the top of your game.

Current Remedies

The choices are vast when it comes to the medical options related to insomnia. Many professionals treat insomnia with prescription medications, such as antidepressants, benzodiazepines, and

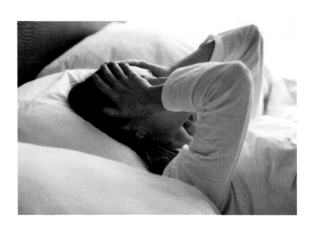

antipsychotics. The problem with that approach is daytime sedation—a hangover effect, as it's called. Curing insomnia with medications can create a host of other problems consistent with dysfunction during waking hours, as well as a long list of side effects. In some studies, many medications have been shown to increase the risk of falls in the elderly and also increase the risk of motor vehicle accidents in people who regularly take medication for insomnia. Sadly, many other solutions are not without risk. Some sufferers self-medicate using over-the-counter (OTC) therapies such as melatonin, valerian, and skullcap, which have some benefits, but most patients do not find them to be as effective as prescription therapies. And some commonly used OTC remedies can be even riskier. The cumulative effect of taking Benadryl® and Zyrtec®, for example, may contribute to the development of memory loss and dementia by decreasing the amount of acetylcholine that our body produces.

Why CBD or Medical Cannabis Might Be the Answer

For those who struggle with sleep, medical marijuana is a medicine that many insomniacs have tried with good results. With the exception of those who suffer from psychosis, medical marijuana (and probably even CBD) has been shown, in a multitude of studies, to aid in the treatment of insomnia without the harsh side effects that prescription and nonprescription drugs induce.

A cannabinoid product with higher levels of Indica seems to be better tolerated by most people, but in a study that provided a questionnaire to some 100 individuals suffering from insomnia and nightmares, high-CBD Sativa strains were reported to be most effective. In a study reported in a 2014 study in the *Journal of Clinical Psychology*, the synthetic product nabilone, mimicking Sativa, was effective in inducing sleep, reducing the frequency of nightmares, and easing chronic pain.

Before selecting any strain of cannabis for long-term use, test various combinations to find the appropriate balance of Indica and Sativa for your personal biological needs. Sleep is often a self-directed journey, so be educated! Also speak to your doctor or dispensary consultant to make sure you're taking the best steps and getting enough support along the way.

SUPPORTING RESEARCH

The endocannabinoid system's CB1 receptors are distributed widely throughout the brain; however, they are absent in the cardio and respiratory centers in the brain stem. This means that while cannabis interacts with brain receptors to help induce sleep and trigger other system repairs, it does not affect heart or pulmonary systems, as do other synthetic drugs. It's safe to consume cannabis without worrying that it will slow your heartbeat or breathing centers, unlike other powerful prescription sedatives and pain relievers.

"I'm a professional yogi, and it's very important that I get a good night's sleep to recover from any of the aches or pains that develop over a day of hard work. At night, I found myself tossing and turning and then waking up at three in the morning, unable to fall back to sleep. A friend suggested trying cannabis, and after getting my medical card, I tried it and had a great sleep, night after night. It's been three weeks now. "

—**Seymour, 48, Yogi**

Integrative Tip > > > > >

When sleep isn't forthcoming and it's hard to settle down after a long day, try lying flat on your back in bed with your face turned slightly to the left or right. Place your hands over your lower abdomen, either side by side with fingertips touching or one on top of the other. Now feel your abdomen rise and fall with your breathing. With each exhalation relax your facial muscles and focus your mind on one important positive personal experience from your busy day. Meditate there to reduce restlessness and fall asleep.

20) Intimacy and Fertility

Intimacy makes the world go round. Not only does it increase the bond between a couple, but it also plays a central role in reproduction. According to couples and parenting expert Mark Banschick, MD, "Sex provides us with a wonderful way to connect with another to experience an ecstatic moment or luxuriate in the sensuality of another body. Intimacy is the experience of true closeness to another, true knowing and being known."

Experts have identified as many as four kinds of intimacy, and not all of them have to do with sex:

- *Experiential intimacy* is the shared feeling between people who may work well together in a club or at work.

- *Emotional intimacy* comes when two people, perhaps siblings, fully entrust their secrets and concerns to each other.

- *Intellectual intimacy* happens when people feel comfortable sharing and discussing ideas no matter how they may disagree.

- *Sexual intimacy* occurs when two people engage in sexual closeness.

Each kind of intimacy can bring people together, but it is sexual intimacy that can forge the closest possible relationship. And this happens by building the relationship on more than physical sex; ideally, it includes all the other forms of intimacy as well. If you can achieve this in your relationship, you'll have found the truest of all partners.

Intimacy is not without its peaks and valleys. Opening one's soul and body to another also sets one up for being vulnerable and potentially getting hurt. Couples in longstanding intimate relationships will tell you that those relationships are worth working for. That's why some of the happiest sexual partners often say, "We were friends first." Once that intimate sharing is in place, it is frosting on the cake to build sexual intimacy to the point where it brings joy to each partner, along with physical and emotional satisfaction.

Working on sexual practice in intimacy can be fun, exciting, and rewarding. Part of it begins with knowing yourself and being able to open yourself to exploring your own and your partner's arousal points, trying new positions, and allowing yourself to slow down and enjoy the experience.

There are challenges to intimacy, of course. In some cases it can be disappointing if a male partner experiences premature ejaculation or erectile dysfunction. A woman's libido may diminish at any age, bringing hypoactive sexual desire disorder (HSDD), which the Society for Women's Health Research has identified as the most common female sexual complaint, experienced by one in ten women. Besides losing the drive for sex, once HSDD begins, orgasm can take longer to reach, last a shorter time, and be less fulfilling. The concern increases with age, along with physical changes, such as vaginal dryness. The good news: You can bring back your libido.

While a certain degree of physical change accompanies age, that doesn't mean sex is off the table. In fact, it can be on the table, on the floor, or anywhere you like, and older couples, especially empty nesters, are rediscovering reckless abandon. Aging gracefully is the key to making it work for you. A softer erection, reduced natural lubrication, or a less intense orgasm doesn't mean you're no longer interested in your partner or in sex itself. For many couples, these kinds of changes only boost their exploration of a new, richer, and every-bit-as-satisfying way to make love—one that's based more on extended foreplay and less on intercourse and orgasm, according to Harvard Health. In these cases, strong emotional intimacy is your lifeline. A survey conducted by AARP (the American Association of Retired Persons) showed that the attributes that make us appealing to a partner—our outlook, shared laughter, and melting eyes—are still ours, and our partners, says the poll, consider them ever more attractive as we age.

Whatever your age, whether you are blossoming and at the forefront of your libido or mellowing and redefining your sexual self, keep in mind that a loving combination of emotional and physical intimacy can bring lasting joy—and it's worth finding ways to enhance it.

Current Treatments

For men, oral medication such as sildenafil (Viagra®) and tadalafil (Cialis®) help correct erection concerns by relaxing the muscles and increasing blood flow in the penis. In cases of prostate surgery or diabetes, other interventions may be more effective, such as a suppository inserted in the urethra or a self-injection at the base of the penis. Penis pumps and inflatable implants are other options. For men experiencing premature ejaculation, a doctor may prescribe a topical anesthetic in cream or spray form with a numbing agent, such as benzocaine, that reduces sensation to delay ejaculation. Antidepressant SSRIs (selective serotonin reuptake inhibitors) and analgesics such as tramadol (Ultram®) may also delay orgasm. Wearing a condom and practicing pelvic floor exercises can help, too.

For women, menopause, pregnancy, breastfeeding, chemotherapy, or removal of ovaries prompt hormonal imbalance, dry vagina, and lower sexual response. In these cases, lubricants, including natural moisturizers—for instance, olive, avocado, or coconut oils—as well as estrogen and other hormone creams that increase blood flow to the vagina may ease sexual interaction and thus pleasure. Estrogen comes in pill, patch, spray, gel, and ring form. Low-dosage estrogen is available in some vaginal creams and slow-releasing suppositories or rings. While estrogen treatment won't help women with HSDD, flibanserin (Addyi™), the first FDA-approved, libido-boosting treatment for premenopausal women, may enhance the sexual experience.

Why CBD or Medical Cannabis Might Be the Answer

More cannabis is used in New York City than in any other city in the United States: Seventy-seven tons a year. That sounds like it's good news for couples in the Big Apple. As a wide array of benefits from marijuana consumption are coming to light in the scientific world, a new study finds that using cannabis can increase the likelihood of intimacy between couples.

As early as 1982, medical studies, first with mice and then with humans, have shown the effect of cannabis on enhancing sexual experience, from increasing desire to prolonging orgasm. A 2007 study published in the *Journal of Psychopharmacology* found that the use of cannabis over alcohol prior to sex led to "a greater perception of interpersonal contact with the partner and a greater willingness to sexually experiment." In 2012, research published in the *Journal of Sexual Medicine* reinforced the relationship between cannabis and arousal in women.

In February 2019, a study titled "Marijuana Use Episodes and Partner Intimacy Experiences" published by the Research Society of Marijuana (RSMj) investigated the impact of cannabis use on couples and whether or not it brought positive effects. In this 30-day study, 183 couples were asked to rate their affection for their partner. It turned out that when couples used cannabis together, they reported a higher rate of lovemaking, affection, and other signs of caring and support.

Similar "significant positive effects" on intimacy were reported when only one partner used cannabis (marijuana) either alone or during intimacy with their partner. "The robust positive effects of using marijuana with one's partner on intimacy events may serve to reinforce continued couple use," the researchers concluded.

One reason for increased intimacy while using cannabis is that cannabis appears to prompt more pleasurable orgasms. A RSMj report published in the *Journal of Sexual Medicine* studied 133 female patients over the age of 18. Three out of four patients exhibited 100 percent improvement in intimacy with the addition of cannabis. Participants reported better overall sexual desire, increased sex drive, and a more pleasurable orgasm with minimal effects on lubrication. In the same journal, a study involving 373 women reported that use of cannabis prompted a two-times-greater likelihood of achieving satisfactory orgasms.

SUPPORTING RESEARCH

Researchers are still determining exactly how cannabinoids enhance libido and sexual enjoyment, but they believe that its role in lowering stress and anxiety opens the door to a more pleasurable sexual experience. Female-based studies have determined that cannabis likely interacts with the pituitary gland to boost the release of sex hormones. Cannabis also interacts with ECS (endocannabinoid system) receptors in the brain to prompt the release of sex-enhancing chemicals like dopamine, which supports sexual excitement in females. Finally, there is a relationship between cannabis and testosterone levels in both males and females, which play a role in sex drive.

Other enhancements to the sexual experience were reported by the *Journal of Sexual Medicine*, observing that cannabinoid use appeared to slow "temporal perception of time and prolong feelings of pleasurable sensations," as well as heighten the senses of touch, smell, taste, sight, and hearing both before, during, and after sex. Finally, cannabis may also help bolster confidence and the desire to experiment.

Dr. Dustin Sulak, founder and medical director of Healer.com and recognized globally in the medical cannabis community, focuses his work on education, advocacy, and research. He explains on Healer.com that "cannabis influences the autonomic nervous system, a major player in sexual attraction, arousal, and orgasm. With inhaled cannabis, most users experience an initial increase in sympathetic [fight-or-flight] nervous system activity, responsible for arousal and ejaculation, followed 15 minutes later by an increase in parasympathetic [rest-and-digest] activity, responsible for erection. The timing of inhaling cannabis before or during a sexual encounter could significantly alter the effects."

But dosage is key, notes Sulak, saying that cannabis can both enhance and interfere with sexual response: "A small dose can be stimulating, while high doses may be too sedating or intoxicating to promote good sex." In fact, a 2019 report in the *American Journal of Men's Health*, which reviewed a decade of studies, notes that it's important for cannabis users—and health-care experts—to under-stand the risk factors for erectile dysfunction when using cannabis.

" I put it [a cannabis-containing lubricant] on and noticed feelings rising in about 10 minutes. I felt a lot of heat and a melting sensation. The arousal hit in a soft kind of gentle wave. Having more than one orgasm never happens, except with cannabis, for me. It happened today! "

—**Stef, 34, Teacher**

Susan Bratton

Susan Bratton is a champion and advocate for all who desire passionate relationships. Considered the "Dear Abby of Sex," Susan's fresh approach and original ideas have helped millions of people of all ages and across the gender spectrum transform sex into passion. Married to her husband Tim since 1993, Susan is an author, award-winning speaker, and serial entrepreneur who teaches passionate lovemaking techniques to her fans around the world. Susan has been featured in *The New York Times* and on CNBC and TODAY. She has also appeared on ABC, CBS, the CW Network, Fox, and NBC as the "Marriage Magician." Susan's straight-talking, fearless approach is rooted in her personal experience of watching her sex life wither while she and her husband pursued dynamic careers. When their relationship hit a crisis point, the couple made a fierce commitment to do whatever it took to keep their family together and revive the passion in their marriage. Today, she and her husband have the kind of dream relationship most people have long-since stopped believing is even possible—until they discover Susan's teachings.

Integrative Tip > > > > >

Honor your most important relationships. Give your close friends and loved ones attention and affection regularly. Placing yourself in a position of service to your friends makes it easy for everyone to count on each other when times are hard.

21) Lung Disease

How many times do you inhale a clear, deep breath and take it for granted? For tens of millions of Americans with asthma, chronic obstructive pulmonary disease (COPD), pulmonary fibrosis, and other pulmonary or lung ailments, taking a deep

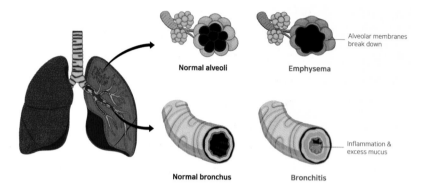

Normal alveoli

Emphysema

Alveolar membranes break down

Normal bronchus

Bronchitis

Inflammation & excess mucus

breath is a luxury. Chronic lower respiratory disease affects people of every age and gender worldwide and is the fourth leading killer in the United States. Our spongelike, air-filled lungs form a beautiful, intricate pulmonary system that works tirelessly, expanding and relaxing thousands of times a day to bring in air with its life-giving oxygen and to expel carbon dioxide as the body's waste. When allergens, infections, smoking, or genetics trigger a glitch in this system, the ability to breathe freely is challenged.

While there are scores of lung diseases, we'll look at some of the more familiar ones. For children in America, the inflammatory condition called asthma is the most common chronic childhood disease. Often related to allergies, asthma can be prompted by household dust and mold, outdoor pollutants, a respiratory infection, or even strenuous exercise. Air passages swell and fill with mucus, and breath becomes short and wheezing, prompting the use of a bronchodilator or other medications to open respiratory passages.

Bacteria or a virus can bring on mild to severe bronchitis or pneumonia; such cases are often acute; that is, they will resolve when any issues are addressed quickly and well. Long-term smokers, however, may develop chronic bronchitis, a condition in which airways become inflamed and a continuous cough produces phlegm. As smoking continues and the disease progresses, it may turn into COPD. In that case, the lungs are so damaged that air cannot easily be exhaled, causing shortness of breath.

Pulmonary fibrosis, another lung disease, may be prompted by environmental toxins or genetics. For an unknown reason, the body begins producing a protein that causes the air sacs in the lungs to stiffen so they can no longer accept air and life-giving oxygen. Lung research is advancing by leaps and bounds, with exciting new therapies that can alleviate all these conditions.

Current Treatments

Asthma patients are usually prescribed a bronchodilator as the frontline tool for opening the airways and arresting an attack. For chronic and severe conditions, a doctor may prescribe inhaled or oral medicines to open air passages, such as over-the-counter fluticasone, or Flonase®, and other stronger medicines. Boosting the immune system through a vegetarian diet and avoiding allergy-inducing milk and eggs often help in the long run, as can massage therapy, acupuncture, yoga, and other moderate, lung-strengthening exercises. Bacterial infections, bronchitis, and pneumonia may be treated with prescription antibiotics. In viral cases, an inhaler and an anti-inflammatory may be prescribed. A humidifier may be used to help loosen mucus from airways. Vaccinations against pneumonia are recommended for at-risk children and adults and for all adults 65 and older. For COPD, the first treatment for a smoker is to stop smoking! In addition—and for nonsmokers—a series of medications may help: An inhaled bronchodilator, such as albuterol, may be prescribed to open airways, or a steroid may help decrease inflammation and prevent acute worsening events, called exacerbations. If another infection, such as bronchitis, sets in, a short-term antibiotic may be needed. Pulmonary fibrosis treatment has recently seen advancements in medications to slow and dissipate fibrosis growth. Two relatively recent FDA-approved drugs have been shown to slow progression: pirfenidone (Esbriet®) and nintedanib (Ofev®). Patients can also work to increase lung capacity through moderate exercise and ongoing breathing therapy.

Why CBD or Medical Cannabis Might Be the Answer

I know just what you're going to ask: How can the inhalation of a smoky product provide any benefit when it comes to reducing respiratory disease?

Actually, it turns out that we have better data on the effects of smoking cannabis on lung health than you might think—and the results may surprise you. In one study published in the journal *Primary Care Respiratory Medicine* in 2016, the effects of cannabis smoking on lung function and respiratory systems were reviewed and, in fact, show that regular use of cannabinoid formulations are associated with an increased forced vital capacity (FVC). If you've ever had to undergo lung testing, this is the portion of the test where the technician asks you to take a deep breath, then exhale as fast and fully as you can, to show how much air you can expel. FVC is a measurement that clinicians rely on to understand the extent of an underlying lung disease, such as COPD or asthma. The stronger the FVC, the healthier the lung.

In a study published in 2013 in the journal *Addictive Behaviors*, researchers found that when tobacco smokers were given the opportunity to use CBD regularly, they were able to reduce their tobacco smoking so effectively that CBD is now being studied rigorously all over the country for its potential use in other addiction scenarios by researchers like Dr. Yasmin Hurd at Mount Sinai Hospital in New York. (See "Addiction and Withdrawal," page 46.)

SUPPORTING RESEARCH

In addition to the importance of FVC as a measure of the extent of a person's lung disease, it is also used to measure how well their body is responding to medications prescribed for the disease. An FVC that has increased after medication is administered is a good sign that the bronchial tubes are dilating in response to the medication and that air is moving well. Studies show that use of cannabinoid formulations can have both bronchodilator and anti-inflammatory effects on the lung. Cannabinoid formulations affect the body's inflammatory pathways in a far different way than do inflammation-producing tobacco products. So much so, in fact, that researchers are testing the addition of cannabinoid formulations and CBD to tobacco products to reduce the amount of inflammation people get from smoking tobacco.

In a study published in 2015 in the journal *Annals of the American Thoracic Society* on the effects of marijuana exposure on expiratory airflow, researchers found that, in a large cross section of US adults, cumulative use of marijuana over a 20-year period showed no adverse changes in functional measures of lung health. Remember: Intense daily use at a very high rate of smoking—regardless of what you're smoking—is going to cause damage. The difference between smoking CBD products or cannabinoid formulations and smoking tobacco cigarettes is this: Smoking a pack of cigarettes per day is equivalent to 250 smoke inhalations a day. Inhaling a dose of cannabinoid formulation might mean only six or seven inhalations a day.

It's also important to remember that when you're smoking cannabinoid formulations, you are getting exposure to terpenes, which are the essential oils of the cannabis plant. Some terpenes, such as pinene, have direct bronchodilator properties; others, such as limonene, offer anti-inflammatory and antibacterial effects. Still others, such as linalool, boost immune system response to infection. The effect of terpenes may explain some of the exciting early studies suggesting that cannabis can actually help lessen the work of breathing and decrease the duration of infection in asthma and bronchitis.

We're going to see some studies in the future that will give us more information on how cannabinoids may help with reducing inflammation.

"My doctor was surprised to see me get almost immediate relief from my asthma attacks after smoking cannabis. The response was just as effective as my inhalers, but without the heart racing and anxiety, unless I selected the wrong strain."

—Debra, 31, Real Estate Agent

Integrative Tip >>>>>
Doing squats every day is one way to increase lung strength and capacity and to keep your hip girdle strong. Being able to stand up and walk unassisted is key to maintaining independence. Every activity that supports strong pelvic girdle muscles will help to keep you healthy and independent as you age, and every activity that

supports strength in the quadriceps, glutes, and lower abdomen involves something similar to a squat. Set a goal for the number of squats you do every day and then have fun trying to figure out how you'll get them in. Sometimes you can do them all in a row, or you can do a few at a time, all day long. For example, I love to do a few squats while I'm waiting for the elevator in my apartment building. I can do five squats taking the elevator down to the main level when I'm bringing my dog out for a walk. Usually I can do ten more squats while I'm walking the dog. Each time I take a break from work to go to the bathroom or get something to drink, I do a few more squats, and, before you know it, I've completed a nice number by the end of the day. Do some with your feet facing straight ahead, but also squat with your toes pointed outward to strengthen the muscles around the knee.

22) Lyme Disease

Summer is tick time. If you're in a wooded area or gardening in a tree-lined backyard, you need to check often for tick bites. No one wants to be among the 30,000 cases of Lyme disease reported yearly by the Centers for Disease Control and Prevention (CDC). Thomas Mather, professor of public health entomology at the University of Rhode Island, has estimated that millions of Americans are bitten by ticks each year. While not every tick bite brings Lyme, it does bring worry. To help allay fears and determine next steps, Mather has established Tick Encounter, a service that connects tick-bite victims to experts. Knowing a few ground rules is key: If you find a tick on your skin, remove it quickly and completely using a pair of tweezers. Keep the specimen in a closed jar, then watch the bite area for the next few days. If a bull's-eye-shaped rash appears, you've likely been infected by *Ixodes scapularis*, commonly known as the deer tick or the blacklegged tick. This tiny vampire, which isn't much larger than a poppy seed, can be identified by its black legs and a roundish black pattern on its back. While drawing blood from deer and other mammals, it picks up a spiral-shaped bacterium, *Borrelia burgdorferi*, which can be transferred when the tick attaches to you. According to CDC experts, the tick needs to be attached for 36 hours to actually transmit the disease; other experts say 24 hours. In any case, it's best not to take chances. Lyme is especially prevalent in the Northeastern and Upper Midwestern United States, where a 2018 study using citizen science participation showed that 50 percent of blacklegged ticks carry the disease. If treated in time, Lyme may resolve with a dose of antibiotics. However, bacteria may lie dormant and return months or even years later, bringing inflammation that triggers chronic fatigue, as well as joint, nervous system, and heart problems. Be on guard: If you notice an expanding rash and experience flulike symptoms, see a doctor.

Current Treatments

Once infected, most patients fully recover after initial treatment with oral antibiotics, such as doxycycline or amoxicillin. In some cases, however, symptoms never completely resolve. Sleep disorders, chronic pain, fatigue, depression, and anxiety may be offshoots that require individualized treatment. As of 2019, the US Food and Drug Administration (FDA) has been reviewing the potential of disulfiram as a potent Lyme disease foe. Also known as Antabuse®, the drug has been approved by the FDA to aid alcoholics in avoiding alcohol. In laboratory studies, however, scientists found that the drug kills not only active Lyme-causing bacteria—the kinds that antibiotics treat—but also other bacteria that resist antibiotics and then lie dormant, later triggering the dreaded chronic symptoms of Lyme. Prevention is always the best frontline medicine: When outdoors, use insect repellent and cover yourself completely. Later, check for ticks in hard-to-see places like the groin, the scalp, and the armpits.

Why CBD or Medical Cannabis Might Be the Answer

As of 2019, the National Institutes of Health (NIH) renewed funding for a clinical study on a new treatment for killing the microbes that cause Lyme. CBD has yet to be studied in such a trial setting as a remedy for Lyme disease. However, its effectiveness in treating the symptoms of pain, bacterial infection, and inflammation that accompany Lyme are well-supported in studies conducted over more than a decade. In 2009, a report in the *Journal of Natural Products* held that many cannabinoids have the potential to guard against tick-borne and other insect-borne bacteria. And a 2012 *Journal of Experimental Medicine* study supports the potential of CBD to "suppress chronic inflammatory and neuropathic pain." A 2018 survey in the journal *Healthcare* noted that the most common symptoms of those conditions are "un-restorative sleep and/or chronic unremitting stress." Both studies open the door for a variety of other conditions that CBD might treat. As a natural neuroprotectant, CBD fortifies the nervous system to ease the stress and anxiety that many report feeling with the disease.

SUPPORTING RESEARCH

Lyme disease is a complicated chronic infection with considerable ongoing chronic inflammation, both in the skin and joints, that also involves the brain and spinal cord. Controlling inflammation and immune response in chronic diseases like Lyme is a very important part of controlling the symptoms of the disease—and cannabis may very well be instrumental in doing just that.

To understand how CBD works, you first need to know about the blood-brain barrier. Although there is some degree of flow between the body and the brain, the blood-brain barrier is in place to protect our precious brains from any unwanted infection or inflammation that may be wreaking havoc elsewhere in the body. Even though the blood-brain barrier appears to slightly weaken with illness, it still poses a challenge for antibiotics or antivirals to cross. In order to address that resistance, it is often necessary to use very high doses of those drugs for long periods of time.

Cannabinoids, however, are known to easily cross the blood-brain barrier. Data show that, just a few minutes after using THC or CBD, symptoms of inflammation, as well as insomnia and anxiety—both conditions affecting the central nervous system—are reduced.

If we know that CBD definitely gets into the brain, the question is this: How can it help? The answer: a lot. First of all, CBD reduces cytokine production. While producing cytokines (the chemicals that give you fever, body aches, and nausea) is the immune system's healthy response to flu or bacterial invaders, too many cytokines can hurt us. CBD helps regulate the production of cytokines to reduce those unwanted symptoms.

Very preliminary data suggest that you can see significant symptom reduction when pretreating with CBD before exposure to colds and flu. And if you're already sick, you can alleviate symptoms when you add CBD to your healing regimen. That's because CBD helps keep cytokines in check and can do the same for Lyme.

Other data gathered over a three-year period on human subjects show how CBD helps modulate the immune system by boosting key immune system warriors: B cells, T cells, natural killer cells, and immunoglobulins—the antibodies that fight infection.

If you're dealing with Lyme or another chronic immune condition, it may be worthwhile to ask your doctor or a cannabinoid expert for their advice on how to use CBD products both to reduce symptoms of the condition and to maintain overall health.

" Cannabis has helped me to get a hold of my gut and skin issues and the anxiety that comes with all of the chronic symptoms that I've been trying to handle with my Lyme disease. I continue to feel the benefits over time. I wake up in the morning and realize I didn't wake in the middle of the night in a panic thinking about my long list of health worries. "

—Charles, 63, Small Business Owner

Integrative (Mandatory!) Tip $>>>>>$
Pull a tick from your skin by grasping its head—not its body—with tweezers and pulling it steadily upward. Grabbing the body risks leaving tick parts behind. Clean the area with rubbing alcohol. You can also remove ticks by waving a match over them or covering them with a thick layer of oil or petroleum jelly. It's important to do a tick check after you've spent any time outside. And remember: Some of these offenders can be tiny in size but mighty in their effect on your health.

23) Metabolic Syndrome

Even if you weren't a cheerleader or a basketball player in high school, you likely weighed less than you do now. Gaining weight is a normal part of aging. Actually, it shouldn't be. The healthiest people in the world maintain just about the same weight through adulthood. And they thank their metabolism for it every day.

Overweight and obesity trigger a cascade of symptoms that include increased waist fat and soaring blood sugar, cholesterol, triglyceride (fat in the blood) levels, and higher blood pressure. These symptoms set the stage for metabolic syndrome—a menacing combo that includes overweight, diabetes, heart disease, and stroke. If you have just one of those conditions, it doesn't mean you have metabolic syndrome. Still, it's a call to action. To find out if you have the condition, work with your physician to do the necessary tests.

You may discover that your blood sugar is unusually elevated. That could signal the onset of diabetes, a condition in which cells are unable to take in sugar from the blood to use as fuel for the body. Cells become starved and tissue is damaged; meanwhile, sugar builds up to dangerous levels in the bloodstream. Blurry vision, fatigue, increased thirst and urination, among other symptoms, result.

Check cholesterol and triglycerides next, to find out how your heart is faring. If your LDL (bad cholesterol) and triglyceride numbers are high while your HDL (good cholesterol) numbers are low, it's likely that plaque is beginning to clog your arteries. (See "Heart Health/Heart Disease," page 90.) Under those conditions, it's harder for blood to circulate around the obstructions, and blood pressure rises. If arteries become completely blocked and blood cannot circulate to your heart or brain, you'll suffer a heart attack or a stroke.

As we age, our susceptibility to metabolic syndrome rises. Watch for these warning signs: weight gain around your abdomen; a family history of diabetes; and your own—or your family's—history of high cholesterol and heart disease. If you suspect that you have metabolic syndrome or any of its components, see your doctor. In the meantime find out all you can about how to achieve the optimal health for your body. Regular exercise and a heart-healthy diet (see the reference to the Mediterranean diet in "Current Treatments" below) are excellent kick-starters.

Current Treatments

Once again, prevention is key. Exercise and a plant-based diet can help you control your weight, cholesterol and triglycerides, and blood pressure.

Both the World Health Organization and US Dietary Guidelines for Americans recognize the Mediterranean diet as sustainable, health-promoting, and preventive for chronic disease. Based on the traditional cuisines of Italy, Greece, and other Mediterranean nations, the diet focuses on fruits, vegetables, whole grains, nuts, and healthy fats, such as olive oil. An integrative diet, it touts exercise, sharing meals with loved ones, and even enjoying a glass of red wine from time to time.

For diabetes patients, a doctor's treatment plan will include checking blood sugar levels throughout the day and may often include taking insulin to keep blood sugar in check. See "Heart Health/Heart Disease," page 90, and "Weight Management," page 141, for other metabolic-related treatments.

Why CBD or Medical Cannabis Might Be the Answer

There are significant wellness markers that link cannabis use with improvement in cardiometabolic risk factors, beginning with a superior waist-to-hip ratio and a lower BMI (body mass index). Regular cannabis smokers just don't seem to gain weight over the years the way other people gain weight after graduating from high school. This capacity to keep a lower "high school body weight" is a very powerful indicator of excellent metabolic health.

Lower body weight is associated with top metabolic outcomes: better high- and low-density lipoprotein cholesterol levels and ratios, lower triglycerides, lower fasting blood sugar, decreased insulin resistance, and lower systolic and diastolic blood pressure, as well as a lower risk of cancer, heart disease, stroke, and other serious common diseases.

While it's likely that much of the benefit to metabolism is achieved through weight control, I suspect that the further direct effects of cannabinoid formulations on metabolism will be clarified in future studies. For instance, research has already shown that, within weeks of starting cannabinoid formulations, patients who did not have significant weight loss did have decreased blood sugar and lower blood pressure. They also had less atherosclerosis and inflammation in their blood vessels and the rest of their body.

Multiple studies conducted on multiple communities around the world have shown both improved metabolism and long-term health and wellness markers linked to cannabis use. In the Inuit population, for example, cannabinoid formulations are shown to reduce obesity and insulin resistance (a marker for the development of diabetes). Other populations that use cannabis regularly have been found to live longer, lead more productive lives, and have very low rates of disease.

SUPPORTING RESEARCH

Researchers previously thought that a plant-based diet, purposeful exercise, a spirituality practice, and maintenance of healthy relationships were the main contributors to human longevity and wellness. Now they are seriously considering the value of cannabis in supporting good health as well. For example, researchers now recognize how cannabis decreases pain and inflammation by interacting with ECS (endocannabinoid system) receptors. Research also shows that, through that interaction, cannabis helps prompt the release of soothing serotonin and dopamine to reduce stress and anxiety. Researchers have only recently come to appreciate that many populations around the world experience less stress, disability, and early mortality because they use cannabinoids as one of their healthy lifestyle practices.

For diabetics, cannabis may turn out to be a potential lifesaver. Researchers have been studying the role of the endocannabinoid system in metabolic syndrome for several decades through both animal models and clinical human trials. Study findings, including those reported in 2019 in the *International Journal of Molecular Sciences*, show that cannabinoids can help block the activation of the CB1R receptor, which is linked to "obesity, insulin resistance, and impaired metabolic function, owing to increased energy intake and storage, impaired glucose and lipid metabolism, and enhanced oxidative stress and inflammatory responses."

Cannabinoid formulations can protect the body from heart disease and stroke by keeping plaques from blocking the arteries. The overwhelming majority of Americans probably have cholesterol plaques in an artery in some part of their body. These arterial plaques need to stay stable and not rupture. If they do rupture and become inflamed, the body will respond by building up a thick layer of platelets—the red blood cells that clot a wound—and macrophages—the white blood cells that fight infection—creating a platelet plug that blocks the artery completely. When blood cannot flow, heart disease and stroke follow. Research reported in 2018 in the *Journal of Microscopy and Ultrastructure* underscores the potential of anti-inflammatory cannabinoids to work as a valuable mechanism to help prevent platelet buildup and protect against heart disease.

When you compare heart disease death rates around the country in maps provided by the CDC (Centers for Disease Control and Prevention), it turns out that areas in the United States where cannabis is legal have much lower death rates from heart disease than those where cannabis use is most restricted. This is also the case with opioid and cancer deaths. For so many reasons, it's time to make cannabis products available to the people who need them.

“*Cannabis has controlled my diabetes. I was diagnosed in October after a long life of eating badly. At 40, I went to the doctor. I was peeing every 10 minutes, I was losing my sight, and my blood sugar was 347. I started smoking a lot of Sativa to get into the right state of mind. In three months, my fasting blood sugar dipped to 100 and I'm diabetes-free. I eat differently and exercise a lot. I do a jailhouse workout because I live in a small apartment.*”

—Terrence, 42, Chauffeur

Integrative Tip >>>>>

Find an excellent salt and use it regularly. Salt is not the health villain it was previously made out to be, and salting your food with an unprocessed salt will replace sodium and other precious minerals lost in sweating and digestion.

24) Multiple Sclerosis (MS)

The National Multiple Sclerosis Society (NMSS) describes multiple sclerosis (MS) as a disease that affects the central nervous system (CNS)—the brain, the spinal cord, and the optic nerves. The body's immune system turns against the CNS, targeting myelin, an insulation around the nerves. Damaged myelin then forms scars, or "sclerosis," giving the disease its name and likely

giving MS its range of symptoms. As MS takes hold, 85 percent of patients experience spasticity (muscle spasms and stiffness). For most, spasticity is mild, but for up to 17 percent of patients, it is severe. Pain is also a common symptom and affects about two-thirds of MS patients. The pain they experience is complex, involving many different chemicals, neurotransmitters, and receptors. In addition, patients can experience various kinds of pain, including headache (43 percent), nerve pain in the arms or legs (26 percent), back pain (20 percent), painful spasms (15 percent), and trigeminal neuralgia (chronic facial pain) (3.8 percent). Most people with MS experience central neuropathic pain caused by damage to the central nervous system or pain from spasms. Inflammation can also cause pain. There is no cure for multiple sclerosis, but there is treatment, which usually focuses on speeding recovery after an attack, slowing the progression of the disease, and managing symptoms. Some people have such mild symptoms that no treatment is necessary.

Current Remedies

Various US Food and Drug Administration (FDA)–approved medications can help reduce the frequency of MS relapses and slow progression of disabilities. Administered orally, through infusions, or by injection, examples include oral

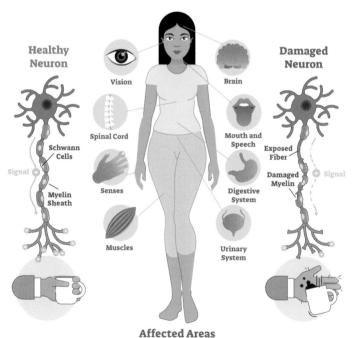

MULTIPLE SCLEROSIS

Healthy Neuron

Vision

Brain

Spinal Cord

Mouth and Speech

Schwann Cells

Signal

Senses

Digestive System

Myelin Sheath

Muscles

Urinary System

Damaged Neuron

Exposed Fiber

Damaged Myelin

Signal

Affected Areas

fingolimod (Gilenya®), injected beta interferons, and infused ocrelizumab (Ocrevus®). Other medications relieve MS symptoms by relaxing muscles; reducing fatigue, depression, and pain; and controlling bladder and bowel incontinence. But none of these medications is completely effective. For instance, although several medications can be used to treat spasticity, they may not work very well, and their use or dose may be limited by side effects. Many people continue to experience relapses, progression, and symptoms from MS.

Why CBD or Medical Cannabis Might Be the Answer

With all the perceived risks of using medical cannabis, limited scientific evidence, concerns about legal status, social stigma, and worries about dependency and the psychoactive effect of getting high, is medical cannabis beneficial in the treatment of symptoms of multiple sclerosis? We can say with certainty, yes! And its use is becoming more common.

Pivotal clinical trials surrounding multiple sclerosis and medical marijuana, which have taken place since 2007, consistently show that cannabis improves certain symptoms and *patients can confidently use CBD and THC to address those symptoms.* A study published in 2011, in an issue of the *European Journal of Neurology*, showed that 75 percent of the participants who used cannabis reported improvements, including better sleep and fewer spasms. Six months after the end of

another study in 2018, 41 percent of the subjects in the study were still experiencing a positive response. In 2017, a survey of MS patients published in the journal *Neurology Clinical Practice* reported that 47 percent of respondents have considered using cannabis, 26 percent have used cannabis, 20 percent have spoken with their physician about using cannabis, and 16 percent are currently using cannabis.

In 2014, the American Academy of Neurology, with some 32,000 neurologists and neuroscientists, published a systematic review of evidence from peer-reviewed journals concerning the "efficacy and safety of medical marijuana in selected neurologic disorders." Conclusions included the following:

- Spasticity reduction: Nabiximols (Sativex® oral spray), oral cannabis extract (OCE), and synthetic THC are probably effective.

- Pain reduction: Nabiximols, OCE, and synthetic THC are probably effective.

- Urinary symptoms: Nabiximols is probably effective for urinary frequency but not for bladder incontinence.

Finally, some very preliminary research suggests that cannabis may also affect the immune system and thus mitigate the immune attacks of MS by decreasing the frequency and intensity of the attacks.

SUPPORTING RESEARCH

In the case of MS, as in many other conditions, two key cannabinoid receptors, CB1 and CB2, are the subjects of ongoing research. CB1 receptors are located primarily in the central nervous system, especially the cerebellum, the basal ganglia, the hippocampus, the cerebral cortex, and the spinal cord, as well as on peripheral nerves. Activation of CB1 receptors is thought to be responsible for the intoxication brought on by the use of cannabis. For instance, while the role of cannabis in MS, and all pain relief, is complex and not well understood, some evidence suggests that CB1 receptors in the brain and peripheral nerves play a role in alleviating pain.

CB2 receptors are located primarily on cells of the immune system and help keep it strong. If chemical neurotransmitters don't interact positively with these receptors, illness occurs. Research shows that THC and CBD may limit inappropriate neurotransmission that leads to MS-related problems.

Studies also show that cannabis may decrease pain by decreasing inflammation.

A Thought on Strains and Products

Two FDA-approved pharmaceuticals are synthetic cannabinoid formulations that mimic THC: dronabinol (Marinol®) and nabilone (Cesamet®). Two oral extracts with THC-to-CBD ratios are not FDA-approved but may be available in marijuana-legal states: nabiximols (Sativex®). Finally, there are botanical cannabis products in different concentrations and proportions of THC and CBD. Typical products in dispensaries have high THC-to-CBD ratios, up to 20:1, but with the growing interest in CBD products, cannabis products with high CBD-to-THC ratios are now available.

> **"** *If I were to sit here right now and focus on the pain from MS, I would not be able to handle it. I went to seven different doctors to manage my pain and remained frustrated and disabled. Finally, the seventh doctor said that many of his patients had gotten relief with medical cannabis and suggested that I give it a try. That was six years ago. Cannabis has controlled my pain and made my life much more livable.* **"**
>
> —Devon, 43, Automotive Industry Executive

Integrative Tip > > > > >

According to the Cleveland Clinic Mellen Center for Multiple Sclerosis, more than 60 percent of MS patients turn to integrative practices to support their pharmaceutical regimen. In addition to a saturated fat–free diet, patients favor reflexology, massage therapy, yoga, meditation, omega-3 fatty acid supplements, acupuncture, Reiki, and tai chi. With those practices, patients not only feel more in control of their disease, their moods lift and they enjoy a greater sense of well-being.

25) Pain (Acute and Chronic)

Pain is personal: Each one of us has a unique experience of it, depending on the kind of pain, the situation in which we experience it, and our memories of how we've dealt with pain in the past.

Pain begins with your spinal cord and brain, where the complex signaling between nerves can be interrupted by any number of daily events and conditions. Basically, a nerve ending is stimulated—perhaps by a cut and tissue damage. In more complex cases, pain results from systemwide damage to nerves, with disruption to their normal signaling—perhaps the result of an old injury or a chronic disease.

There are two kinds of pain: acute and chronic. *Acute* pain is brought on by a specific incident, such as a knife nick or a stove burn in the kitchen, a broken arm from falling off a bike, a sunburn at the beach, a pulled muscle after a game of tennis, or even a hearty sneeze! By addressing such incidents quickly and efficiently, you can ease pain over a period of days or weeks and restore your body's equilibrium.

Chronic pain, on the other hand, does not have an easy fix. Often defined as lasting more than 12 weeks, chronic pain can persist for months and even years. Also, it may leave painful aftereffects that continue to haunt you long after an acute injury or infection has healed. Aging is often the culprit behind chronic pain: The wear and tear of life may bring unrelenting back and muscle aches or knees swollen with arthritis. Certain conditions such as migraine, irritable bowel syndrome, multiple sclerosis, and cancer can cause chronic pain and can be even harder to bear if the pain is aggravated by your surroundings—perhaps a polluted environment—or even your personal outlook.

Neuropathic pain is chronic pain that typically arises from damage to the nervous system from either blunt force trauma such as a motor vehicle accident, from a direct injury, or from a pinching or stabbing wound. Sometimes neuropathic pain is prompted by an internal pinching, such as a slipped disc. It's also associated with many diseases like multiple sclerosis, where nerve pain is caused by demyelination (damage to the protective covering that surrounds nerve fibers), or Parkinson's disease, HIV, diabetes, and also, unfortunately, as a consequence of chemotherapy for patients who have survived cancer.

In addition, there are several debilitating, severe chronic pain syndromes. One of the most debilitating is complex regional pain syndrome (CRPS), once called reflex sympathetic dystrophy syndrome (RSD), which is characterized by chronic severe pain that appears to be much greater than the pain inflicted by the initial injury. The affected area might be highly sensitive and swollen, with changes in skin quality.

In general, older adults experience more chronic pain due to the prevalence in this age group of cancer, arthritis, diabetes, heart disease, or neurological conditions. Pain may also be brought on simply by aging. Research shows that women experience more chronic pain than men and may experience two or more chronic pain conditions.

While pain is personal, how we treat it is personal, too. Chronic pain can cause depression and social isolation, creating more pain in a vicious cycle. The first step toward treating pain is to identify how it affects you. Basic pain medications—whether over-the-counter or prescription—may help for a while, but stronger, more targeted medications may be required. To help any medicine work to its max, be sure to build a healing integrative program for yourself that includes physical therapy, exercise, plenty of sleep, and a healthy diet. A healthy lifestyle will open doors to long-term management of chronic pain. Remember to keep your social networks strong. Family, friends, a trusted therapist—all are waiting to help. And sometimes helping someone whose need is even greater than yours is the most effective pain reliever of all.

Current Treatments

Motrin® (ibuprofen) is terrific for localized pain because it works through prostaglandin pathways to reduce painful prostaglandin production. The way Motrin works is totally different from the way cannabinoids impact neurotransmitters at the transmitting sites. You could always use Motrin in combination with cannabis to see if you can get any additional relief from pain. If you have any type of opiate available, you could also try that, probably at quite a lower dose than you've tried before.

Don't forget about heat and ice. Most doctors recommend icing after an acute trauma or if the pain has increased due to an overuse injury typical of weekend warrior syndrome, which occurs when people overdo activities on the weekend, resulting in more pain or even a new injury. Injuries respond well to ice, but generally after a period of acute trauma (about 12 to 24 hours), it's more beneficial to apply a heating pad because the heat dilates the blood vessels and helps bring more healing blood flow to the injured, painful area.

Sometimes it can help to confuse pain receptors by using a combination of ice and heat. Blasting the affected area with a very cold ice pack, followed by a warm heating pad, will make it hard for pain receptors to sense the pain. This method can sometimes do a nice job of easing pain before you go to bed.

Also think about using a brace instead of a bandage for a joint that's unstable or if you need to limit the range of motion in the joint to reduce your pain. Don't wear a brace when you are resting or lying in bed, however, as it can restrict blood flow. Finally, consider physical therapy or massage to help alleviate pain. If you don't have a chiropractor, a physical therapist, a personal trainer, or a yoga teacher on your pain team, find one. They will bring the appropriate stretching and flexibility training to the table to help you get better and bring pain under control as much as possible.

Neuropathic pain is notoriously difficult to treat. We've tried all kinds of different medications to address the issue, and perhaps you've tried some of them yourself. For example, we use antidepressants in an attempt to bump up serotonin, to help decrease the anxiety and depression associated with pain, as well as reducing the painful syndrome within the central nervous system. We also use gabapentin, a medication also known by the brand name Neurontin®, that works to impact the GABA receptors in your brain and reduce pain through that pathway. Seizure medications are also used to reduce chronic pain by decreasing the painful stimulus from interacting with other cells around it.

Sometimes when you burn a finger, the injury may affect only the tip, but the rest of your hand feels a little hypersensitive as well. That's because when the information that the tip of your finger has been hurt travels to the brain, a lot of other cells in your finger become inflamed and irritated, too, and start responding to the stimulation in the area. Seizure medications and sometimes antidepressants will help reduce that response and limit the amount of pain from that stimulus. Sometimes seizure medications can be effective in addressing neuropathic pain, but, as I've discovered and as you may know from personal experience, there are limitations to these medications, and none of them manages pain very well.

Besides medicines, whether they're pharmaceuticals or cannabis, you might consider other valuable therapies, such as acupuncture, biofeedback, and stretching and flexibility with a good physical therapist, yogi, personal trainer, orthopedist, or any other person who can help give your muscles and your skeleton better support. In cases of fibromyalgia, rheumatoid arthritis, osteoarthritis, and other generalized pain syndromes, we've previously recommended stretching, massage, and exercise, while recognizing the limitations of those methods for people who are in pain.

Why CBD or Medical Cannabis Might Be the Answer

If you're dealing with an area of focused, localized pain in your neck, knee, elbow, or shoulder, for example, consider using a CBD balm or tincture. These excellent pain relievers are applied locally and topically by rubbing them into the affected area. These relievers also work well when combined with Motrin or with a heat and ice treatment (see page 122). Be sure to combine CBD with other medicines only under a doctor's supervision.

Some balms are made with aromatics that have medicinal properties, such as eucalyptus for muscle relaxation and lemon for energy. Consider alternating a medicinal herbal balm with a high-CBD-containing product or alternate a high-CBD product with a low-THC product (between 9 percent and 15 percent CBD) to help alleviate pain.

In the case of chronic pain, medical marijuana may offer a terrific opportunity to help you feel better. In cases of fibromyalgia, rheumatoid arthritis, osteoarthritis, and other generalized pain syndromes, it has been shown to be helpful,

beyond stretching and massage, as noted in "Current Treatments" (page 121). You'll be excited to hear about the Israeli study published in the *Journal of Clinical Rheumatology* in February 2018. The 36 participants in the study had chronic pain from underlying musculoskeletal conditions and were asked to respond to a pain questionnaire before and after being treated with medical marijuana over a 10- to 11-month period.

Amazingly, all 36 patients reported improvements in their pain. Only 30 percent reported adverse events, which were mild and didn't result in the discontinuation of their treatment with marijuana. Astonishingly, half the patients discontinued the baseline prescription medication they had been using and continued to use only medical marijuana to treat their pain.

There's a really nice study published in 2011 by the *British Journal of Clinical Pharmacology* that gives us some hope that cannabis could be a valuable treatment for chronic neuropathic pain syndromes. The study reviewed 18 individual studies that focused on the use of cannabis to manage pain. Fifteen of the studies showed that the participants saw improvement in pain. They also reported improvement in the quality of their sleep and no serious adverse effects from their treatment. Those results led the researchers to conclude that the use of medical marijuana or cannabis for neuropathic pain should be considered safe and moderately effective for pain management, in addition to the seizure medications, antidepressants, or other pharmacological therapies that a patient many be using.

Another study, published in 2018 by *La Clinica Terapeutica* involved 338 patients who were treated with medical marijuana for 12 months to address chronic pain stemming from various disorders. First, the patients filled out a questionnaire regarding their pain medications, the intensity of their pain, the level of their disability, and the amount of anxiety and depression they were experiencing in association with their pain. The patients were then requestioned at months 1, 3, 6, and 12. A significant number of the patients reported reductions in pain intensity, reductions in pain disability, and reductions in anxiety and depression.

There are some significant limitations to this study, however. For one, the type of pain used for baseline assessment wasn't a specific type, and there was no control group. Still, the study led researchers to conclude that patients might experience significant alleviation of chronic pain with the addition of medical marijuana to a treatment protocol.

SUPPORTING RESEARCH

To help treat pain, a product high in CBD—or perhaps even pure CBD—will help relax the muscles and also boost serotonin levels. A bit of THC might be helpful: Adding a low amount of THC to the CBD may enhance muscle relaxation and also address anxiety and depression. But be careful. Too much THC may limit the pain-relieving effects of the CBD, which is the gold standard in anxiety and depression management. The more THC there is in a product, the less anxiety control a patient will have, along with less muscle relaxation. A high-CBD, low-THC-ratioed medical marijuana product appears to be most useful. By holding the tincture in your mouth for a minute or so before swallowing, you'll allow the product to cross through the mucus membranes and potentially speed the absorption of the formulation.

A Thought on Strains and Products

I would consider choosing a hybrid product that's a little bit heavier on the Sativa end. That's because most people who are dealing with chronic neuropathic pain also deal with a lot of fatigue—and having a higher level of energy with a higher concentration of Sativa in the hybrid would be ideal. There are various benefits of using a Sativa as opposed to an Indica hybrid. A good direction to follow on your first try may be something high in CBD, possibly from a Sativa-containing plant. See if you can get some relief from it. I'd love to hear your success stories.

> **❝** *Cannabis makes me feel very fluid and always has; I think it opens everyone up, both physically and mentally. I've used it for six years now for my arthritis pain, with no side effects, and I'm not addicted to opiates like a lot of my friends who suffer with similar pain.* **❞**
>
> —**Carl, 76, Retired, Air Force**

Integrative Tip $>>>>>$

Eat the garnish on your plate! Don't let that precious dark leafy green serving go back to the kitchen and land in the trash. Dark-green leaves are the most nutrient-dense foods available.

26) Parkinson's Disease

Symptoms of Parkinson's disease begin with lack of muscle control. A person may feel a tremor in a hand, which may progress to both hands and then to their arms, legs, and head.

Here's what scientists know: Parkinson's disease (PD) is a degenerative, progressive disorder that affects nerve cells (neurons), in deep parts of the brain called the basal ganglia and the substantia nigra. In the substantia nigra, the neurons produce the neurotransmitter dopamine, which sends messages to the body, controlling our movements. In Parkinson's patients, these cells begin to die and dopamine is no longer produced. Stiffness, tremor, slowed gait, and balance issues ensue.

Scientists are still determining what prompts this death of cells. While Parkinson's may run in families, it may also be the result of environmental toxins or another severe disease like encephalitis. As it progresses, it may be accompanied by non–motor-related symptoms, such as depression, constipation, insomnia, diminished sense of smell, and dementia. While Parkinson's itself is not fatal, these and other disease complications may be serious. According to the Centers for Disease Control and Prevention (CDC), Parkinson's is the fourteenth leading cause of death in the United States.

As of yet, there is no cure for Parkinson's, but there are hopeful treatments, from medications to surgeries. Following a physician's guidance and recommended therapies are key. With awareness of the disease, its progression, and its treatments, patients can enjoy a robust quality of life for many years.

Current Treatments

Parkinson's is generally treated with dopaminergic drugs, which address the low levels of dopamine in the brain due to impairment of neurons in the substantia nigra.

Current prescription medications, such as the benzodiazepine clonazepam induce sedation at bedtime, which can last well into the daytime. This can increase the risk of falls and motor vehicle accidents, especially in the elderly, making CBD a safer alternative for those who are prone to accidents.

Surgery is another option. Scientists are exploring ways to identify biomarkers for PD that can lead to earlier diagnosis and more tailored treatments to slow down the progress of the disease. Currently, all therapies used for PD improve symptoms without slowing or halting its progression.

Why CBD or Medical Cannabis Might Be the Answer

Can patients with Parkinson's disease benefit from CBD or medical cannabis? The research says yes. It can actually help patients get a better night's sleep. Although there isn't much research surrounding the use of CBD and cannabis for Parkinson's disease, one particular study caught my eye. In a 2014 edition of the *Journal of Clinical Pharmacy and Therapeutics*, case reports reviewed the sleep disorders of six patients with Parkinson's disease. One patient, a 61-year-old man, had developed rapid eye movement (REM) sleep behavior disorder (RBD), in which he had nightmares that brought on violent reactions, such as punching, kicking, and yelling. After six weeks of taking CBD, he and the other participants saw a full reversal of RBD. Researchers think that CBD, or CBD combined with THC, will be beneficial in increasing the duration of REM sleep (the period when dreaming occurs in the sleep cycle) for patients with RBD.

In a 2018 article in the journal *Frontiers in Integrative Neuroscience*, neuroscientist and cannabis luminary Ethan B. Russo, MD, reported that an observational study showed that 22 out of 28 PD patients who smoked cannabis "showed acute benefits on tremor, rigidity and bradykinesia (slowness of movement)." Russo also noted that CBD was helpful in treating five PD patients with psychosis.

In addition, CBD has been shown in rat models to have neuroprotective benefits against Parkinson's. In fact, in 1998, a US patent based on the health benefits of CBD as an antioxidant was filed by the National Institutes of Health (NIH). Among the benefits discussed, the top was neurodegenerative disease protection. Ongoing tests by independent research laboratories are evaluating the role of high-grade CBD oil in reducing oxidative stress and the formation of free radicals, which break down healthy cells. Ongoing modulation of inflammation and oxidative stress is possible with the administration of CBD oil.

SUPPORTING RESEARCH

Parkinson's disease has long been attributed to the death of neurons in certain parts of the brain, such as the basal ganglia and the substantia nigra. These neurons produce the neurotransmitter dopamine, which sends out messages controlling body movement. When dopamine is no longer produced, tremor, slowed movement, stiffness, and impaired balance set in. In some cases, these neurons may develop a protein-based fibroid—the same kind that occurs in Alzheimer's patients, impairing the release of dopamine. In the same 2018 article in *Frontiers in Integrative Neuroscience* cited above, Dr. Russo wrote that nabiximols (Sativex®), a cannabis extract that has not been approved yet by the FDA (US Food and Drug Administration), reduces this fibroid buildup "with improvement in dopamine metabolism . . . as well as reducing anxiety and self-injury."

NIH-supported studies in 2012 and 2014 showed that CBD helped reverse cognitive decline in rats treated with iron, a promising development for patients with Alzheimer's disease and Parkinson's disease who suffer from motor and cognitive impairment (such as memory loss) due to the buildup of iron in the brain. CBD also helped clean out accumulated proteins and other particles that can trigger fibroid buildup and cell death. And Parkinson's patients in a 2014 trial, published by the journal *Psychopharmacology*, reported improved quality of life and relief of tremors and other symptoms after a course of CBD.

To help Parkinson's patients sleep, look to the CB1 receptors in the brain, which are thought to regulate the sleep/wake cycle. The endocannabinoid anandamide stimulates these receptors during sleep, increasing the length of slow-wave and REM sleep. With chemical structures similar to anandamide, CBD and THC can help the body react in the same way, promoting a deeper, more nourishing sleep pattern. With the addition of CBD to their healing regimen, Parkinson's patients can finally get a good night's sleep!

> "*Cannabis calms me down immediately. Using just a small amount of tincture, my hands are rock steady and there's no dyskinesia. It makes me angry that I can't get it in my home state.*"
>
> **—Neely, 56, Publicist**

Dr. Greg Eckel

Dr. Greg Eckel has spent the last 20 years developing and refining his unique approach to chronic neurological conditions. In addition to using a combination of naturopathic and traditional Chinese medicine, he has a deep personal connection with chronic neurological disease: His wife Sarieah passed away from Creutzfeldt-Jakob disease (CJD), a condition with no known cure. She was the love of his life, and in her name he took a deep dive into research, soon developing a brain-regenerative program to help patients with neurological conditions improve their quality of life and find natural solutions. An internationally recognized speaker and the author of *Shake it Off: An Integrated Approach to Parkinson's Solutions*, he is cofounder and owner of Nature Cures Clinic in Portland, Oregon.

High-antioxidant foods and supplements may help to reduce the oxidative burden in the brain and slow loss of brain function in Parkinson's. Antioxidants can be derived from fruits growing deep within the Amazon rain forest, but they can also be found in far less exotic, less expensive, and just-as-effective fruits, vegetables, and dark leafy greens that grow a lot closer to home. The USDA's list of top 20 foods high in antioxidants includes a range of choices, from red kidney beans, cranberries, and artichokes to strawberries, pecans, red delicious apples, and, of course, dark leafy greens.

27) Post-Traumatic Stress Disorder (PTSD)

I'd like you to take a look at somebody near you right now. Or, better yet, take a look in the mirror. Can you tell by looking at someone whether or not they've suffered a severe traumatic event in their life? I can't, either. Post-traumatic stress disorder is defined as an anxiety disorder stemming from a severe physical injury or severe emotional stress. I can't tell by looking at somebody whether they've had a traumatic event, but when I talk to them and start to dig deeper, I can see it in all the other conditions that arise from chronic stress, like anxiety and depression, obesity, chronic fatigue, and increased risk of heart attack, stroke, and other metabolic conditions.

The brain doesn't distinguish between good and bad information. It's just a sponge, gathering all the information that's nearby. But when it experiences a bad situation, the brain isn't really disordered—and, in fact, I take issue with the name *post-traumatic stress disorder*. It really should be called post-traumatic stress *reorder*, because that brilliant brain of yours reorders under stress, and the neural tissues restructure so that you can survive the trauma you're enduring.

The prefrontal cortex, which is usually in charge of applying logic to emotion, does not work as effectively under stressful situations; consequently, the brain functions in a much more primal and emotional way. The hippocampus, which is usually in charge of storing short-term memory, also becomes less effective under stress, resulting in changes in the brain's ability to modulate the logical response to emotion and reducing its capacity to store short-term memory. The amygdala functions as a little general and commands the hypothalamus and the pituitary gland to release a ton of stress hormones. Those glands and parts of the brain then generate responses within the adrenal glands, the thyroid gets activated, and suddenly your entire body is in fight-or-flight mode, preparing you either to fight whatever you're facing or to run away from it.

This hyperarousal syndrome sticks around for quite a while. But after the initial adverse event, as you receive additional stimuli that cause smaller arousals, you can develop a sensitized sensory pathway. Suddenly, very small triggers result in tremendously significant responses.

Patients suffering from PTSD are hypervigilant and develop avoidance techniques to stay away from situations that can prompt a flashback and the anxiety that comes with it. They also have intrusive thoughts with graphic images, and their sleep is riddled with nightmares. Overall, life is distressing, and managing symptoms is crucial.

Current Remedies

Medications that help with depression and anxiety can also help with PTSD. Lexapro®, Zoloft® and Buspar are a few. But side effects, such as tremors and insomnia, are common with these medications. However, there are also exciting new trends in ancient herbal therapies, such as cannabis, that are proven to be very effective for this condition when combined with modern medicine or when used independently. Beyond medicines, extinction therapies are helping reduce symptoms. Like Pavlov's dogs, who were trained to salivate for food when a bell rang, PTSD patients can be trained into and out of a fear response. This gives hope to PTSD patients suffering from terror-ridden responses to a stimulus. That response can be reduced through repeated exposure therapy in which the patient keeps getting the exposure but not the same conditioned experience. Instead, the new experience is one that evokes a happy memory. This counter-conditioning helps a patient associate a response with a happy memory and thus terminate the usual bad response. We also know that we can help the body relax through massage and exercise, to send positive signals back to the brain. We've also used plenty of great medications for this condition. Working with the right health-care professionals, using every potential tool that's available, including cannabis, can help you get better faster and live a really effective, really beautiful, whole life.

Why CBD or Medical Cannabis Might Be the Answer

Does regular use of cannabidiol help people with PTSD? In a 2017 study published in the *Journal of Abnormal Psychology*, researchers looked at patients who were suffering from anxiety and who were either nonusers or chronic users of cannabidiol. When exposed to loud noises, the patients were checked for their response—whether their hair stood on end or they broke out in a sweat. In attempting extinction treatment to fully wipe out those responses, researchers found that patients who used cannabidiol either daily or at least five times a week could not be treated as effectively as nonusers in the study. This finding seems to run counter to what we have learned from animal studies, which show that stimulating CB1 receptors during treatment—not on a daily basis— actually improves treatment. However, animal studies also show that chronic, routine daily use of cannabidiols can result in decreased efficacy of treatment.

So why recommend daily use of cannabidiols? An extinction study in 2013 showed that while it was not effective during the study, subjects showed a sustained positive response when using cannabidiol afterward. And, while cannabidiol may not effect "extinction" of PTSD, it helps manage accompanying symptoms that can be debilitating and increases overall well-being. Cannabidiol does this by stimulating the CB1 receptors on an ongoing basis, quelling anxiety, insomnia, and more—helping people who are disabled by their experience to establish stability in their lives. For instance, it helps keep stable levels of the chemical cortisol, which can soar out of control during a PTSD episode, increasing blood pressure, interfering with memory, and prompting extreme anxiety. From 2012 to 2015 a study carried out across Canada, the United States, Mexico, and Israel showed that through ongoing cannabidiol use, people with PTSD not only had lower anxiety and better sleep but also fewer intrusive thoughts.

SUPPORTING RESEARCH

The endocannabinoid (ECS) system is already involved in managing stress and controlling memory. Its CB1 receptors, which are abundant in the brain, especially in the prefrontal cortex and the hippocampus, can help make situations emotionally understandable and contextualize them with past experiences so that the stress response and anxiety are controlled. Evidence shows that reduced functionality within the ECS—that is, lower ECS tone—may predispose a person to PTSD. In a 2001 study following the World Trade Center attacks, it was found that subjects with decreased anandamide—the most common endocannabinoid—were at highest risk for developing PTSD.

Endocannabinoids, the body's own THC and CBD, help reduce anxiety and depression while also helping to build new memories and replace old, unsettling ones. They also support neuroplasticity, the optimal communication between neurons, to help change patterns of communication within the brain so as to establish a new, safe response to trauma.

"After military service I came home, and six months later I had stopped taking care of myself. I had really bad anxiety. I was hypervigilant and had to face the door when I was in restaurants. I eventually stopped leaving the house. Fear permeated everything. Initially I was diagnosed with personality disorder, but eventually they figured out it was PTSD and I was given medications through the VA for pain and anxiety. They left me feeling sedated. I saw a PBS special about how medical cannabis helped veterans. I asked one of my friends to get me some weed, and we smoked a joint in my living room. We laughed and joked. The pills helped me to not feel anything, but the cannabis made me think. Now I have a cannabis community and even though I still have a hard time, I'm doing better."

—**Trevor, 38, Television Production Assistant**

Dr. Keesha Ewars

Dr. Keesha Ewars is a board-certified functional and Ayurvedic medical practitioner, a doctor of sexology, a family practice ARNP (advanced registered nurse practitioner), a certified psychotherapist, a huachumera (medicine woman trained in the use of plant medicine from Peru), a Reiki master, and an angel therapist trained by Doreen Virtue. Dr. Ewars is the founder of a new branch of medicine called functional sexology. She is also the founder and a host of the Healthy YOU! Radio Network. Dr. Ewars practices what she calls "mystic medicine," where *everything* is seen as God, including illness and suffering. "Once that lesson is learned," she teaches, "the struggle is relieved." She helps people to release trauma from childhood and beyond and to find lasting peace.

Integrative Tip >>>>>
When facing a stressful situation, stop for a moment and mindfully take 10 deep breaths in and out. You're engaging the vagus nerve, which then signals the nervous system to slow your heart rate, lower your blood pressure, and decrease your cortisol level. Within seconds you'll feel your body relax.

28) Psychological Conditions (Bipolar Disorder [Manic Depression] and Schizophrenia)

While anxiety and depression are conditions of the mind that can cause seemingly endless worry and darkness, more serious psychological conditions can bring even deeper concerns. Bipolar disorder (formerly called manic depression) is one of them. About 2–3 percent of the global population who live with the condition experience debilitating symptoms that affect energy levels,

activity, and mood, which can swing dramatically from emotional highs (mania) to extreme lows (depression), sometimes on rare occasions or several times a year. Such changes may be due to periods of high stress or a traumatic experience, such as a car accident or the loss of a loved one. Under those circumstances, sleep, activity, judgment, and the ability to think clearly are affected. The causes of bipolar disorder are as uncertain as the cure, but medications and therapy are available and researchers are working toward a remedy that can help restore balance and quality of life to those who suffer from this serious condition.

Schizophrenia is an incurable, chronic condition in which daily reality becomes distorted. A person's thoughts and speech may be jumbled, and they may hear voices and hallucinate, act irrationally, exhibit paranoia, be combative and aggressive; and basically ride an emotional roller coaster. It goes without saying that it's almost impossible to function in society with this condition. Lifelong treatment is necessary to help put the symptoms into remission, but they can resurface at a moment's notice. Schizophrenia may be triggered by family history, brain chemistry, toxic chemical exposure, or early drug use. In severe cases, hospitalization is needed. Uncontrolled schizophrenia may lead to depression, social isolation, health and financial problems, homelessness, and even suicide.

Current Remedies

Antipsychotic medications are the first line of defense for schizophrenia. Most interact with the brain neurotransmitter dopamine to control symptoms. Recent medications on the market, such as aripiprazole (Abilify Maintena®), asenapine (Saphris®), and brexpiprazole (Rexulti®), have fewer side effects than the antipsychotic drugs that were used in the past. Drugs for bipolar disorder include mood stabilizers, such as lithium, benzodiazepine antianxiety medications, antipsychotics (risperidone), antidepressants, and drugs that act both as antipsychotics and as antidepressants. Bipolar disorder is a sensitive condition with a number of different triggers. Don't forget that a lot of products have also been linked to triggering mania, including Western medications used to treat depression, like bupropion and trazodone, as well as herbal therapies like Saint John's wort, ginseng, horny goat weed, and celery root, to name just a few.

Why CBD or Medical Cannabis Might Be the Answer

Of the 2.3 million Americans who suffer from bipolar disorder, many have found significant improvement in their condition when using cannabis or other cannabinoid products. Several trials have backed this up. Patient reports are abundant: Not only do many of them feel better, but they are also better able to manage their behavior. When you look at the extent and the thoroughness of the research, it's clear that the use of cannabinoids will generally result in improved mood and better behavior. Study results in an article published in 2016 by the journal *PLOS ONE* found that patients with bipolar disorder who regularly smoked cannabis reported at least short-term mitigation of symptoms, indicating "potential mood-stabilizing properties."

However, there are concerns that cannabis could potentially harm short-term memory and executive function, which includes the ability to perform a series of cognitive tasks to problem-solve effectively. Those concerns arise more often when cannabis is taken for other conditions and don't seem to have the same level of impact in the bipolar community. In fact, the 2016 *PLOS ONE* report found that cannabis use did not impair cognition in patients who participated in the study.

There have also been reports that synthetic THC has actually triggered mania in people with a history of bipolar disorder. That's something to worry about. It would suggest that if you're going to use cannabinoids for bipolar treatment, it's preferable to use products higher in CBD and lower in THC, so there is less risk of hyperstimulating the brain. Don't forget that a lot of other products have also been linked to triggering mania, like those mentioned previoulsy, in "Current Remedies."

For bipolar disorder, a sensitive condition with different treatments, we have limited data on how cannabis formulations can be used to help address the condition. As of 2020, an ongoing 30-year review of at least 47 studies, published in the *American Journal on Addictions*, is assessing our current clinical understanding of cannabis for treating bipolar and related conditions and where we need to go from here. The overarching view, however, looks very reassuring.

SUPPORTING RESEARCH

In schizophrenia and bipolar disorder, it appears that physical changes in the structure of the brain and nervous system are features of both conditions. Because the endocannabinoid system (ECS) works as a mood regulator, it's feasible that it could step in to help both. The ECS creates the endocannabinoid anandamide, which works with CB1 and CB2 receptors to enhance mood. If the ECS can't supply the amount of anandamide that is needed, studies show that the cannabinoids THC and CBD, which have similar chemical structures to anandamide, can. But too much can actually boost schizophrenic symptoms. In the case of schizophrenia, psychiatric researchers at New York University's Langone Medical Center have found that cannabis with higher concentrations of CBD can reduce the risk of developing psychotic disorders and keep the brain from experiencing cognitive changes related to the disease. A study on schizophrenic patients, published in a 2018 issue of the *American Journal of Psychiatry*, used CBD to supplement regular antipsychotic medication and found that CBD users saw significant improvement, compared to a placebo group. How the ECS is linked to bipolar disorder is still in the early stages of discovery. But because of the ECS's role in mood control, researchers, as of 2019, were looking into how activation of the CB2 receptor might stabilize mood. We do know that cannabis products have an impact on the depression that accompanies bipolarism's "low" and on the anxiety that can come with its "high." (See "Depression," page 70, and "Anxiety," page 53.)

" The Trileptal® controlled the bipolar, but it also took away so many of my emotions; it left me flat, rather than joyful or sad, and I gained 150 pounds. Careful selection of the right cannabis—I didn't want to make things worse— has been a godsend for me. It's completely controlled my symptoms. I can adjust it as needed during times when I'm feeling the mania coming on or if I'm activating it myself by working too much. Most important, I feel like myself again after 18 years of feeling like a zombie. "

—Agnes, 56, Editor

Integrative Tip > > > > >

Exercise helps many people relax and can also be a good time to meditate. Replace sedentary time sitting in front of the TV with exercise to help strengthen your muscles and get the stretching and flexibility you need without having to carve out extra time from your busy schedule to travel to a gym.

29) Skin Conditions

Soft as a silk; tough as armor. That's your skin—the largest organ in your body. Every day it cleanses your system of internal and environmental toxins and blocks invading microorganisms. As the gateway to your inner sanctum, skin touched by the sun delivers vitamin D to regenerate cells and to build strong bones and other organs.

You need to treat it right. Exercise, especially outdoors, improves circulation to keep skin in the pink. Getting regenerative sleep, lowering stress and practicing well-being, filling up with antioxidant fruits and vegetables, and drinking cleansing water all contribute to healthy skin.

Even the most skin-conscious among us is exposed to daily pollution, poisonous plants, toxic cleaning chemicals, stress and anxiety, lack of sleep, and poor food, all of which can incite dermatitis, a condition in which the skin becomes inflamed.

Atopic dermatitis, also called eczema, often begins in infancy and sometimes occurs where skin flexes, inside elbows or behind knees; contact dermatitis comes from interaction with poison ivy, cleaning chemicals, and even nickel-containing jewelry; seborrheic dermatitis, caused by a yeast in the skin's oil secretions, causes cradle cap and, later, dandruff.

Skin rash can be unsightly and uncomfortable, with itchy, weeping, crusty patches. Dryness, redness, flaking, blistering, cracking, or bleeding may be part of the condition. Do not scratch open a healing lesion—you'll either infect the rash, make it bigger, or both.

Other causes of dermatitis include radiation during cancer treatment, seasonal allergies, or an allergic reaction to food that may cause hives—small, red, itchy bumps.

Psoriasis is a condition in which the skin produces new cells faster than they can be sloughed off. The result is a pileup of plaques (raised red patches) on the skin that show up primarily on the scalp, elbows, knees, and buttocks. Infection, stress, tobacco smoke, and dietary gluten can all be triggers. While there is no cure for this chronic disease, medications and lifestyle changes can go a long way toward helping to manage it.

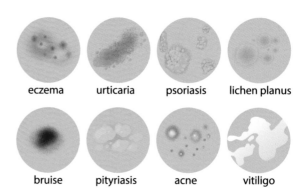

eczema   urticaria   psoriasis   lichen planus

bruise   pityriasis   acne   vitiligo

And then there is acne, a teenage and, sometimes, adult nightmare that occurs when hair follicles fill with oil from sebaceous (oil) glands and become infected, mainly on the face, shoulders, chest, and back. Hormones, medications, stress, and diet all may play a part in triggering acne.

In all cases, practice skin health: Shower quickly in warm water (hot water dries out skin), ditch cigarettes (smoking depletes oxygen and nutrients), use a moisturizer with a high SPF daily to guard against harmful ultraviolet rays, get plenty of sleep, and eat well.

Current Remedies

Prescription corticosteroid ointments, creams, and gels can go a long way toward soothing the symptoms of dermatitis and psoriasis. Also, a topical medication called calcineurin helps reduce itching and inflammation by interacting with the immune system. Controlled phototherapy (light therapy) helps, too. A simple recommendation is to use a daily moisturizer to lock in moisture and reduce dryness, scaling, and itching. In the case of psoriasis, over-the-counter salicylic acid promotes removal of dead skin cells to limit scaling. Also, synthetic vitamin D creams, such as calcipotriene (Dovonex®), help to slow skin cell growth. In severe cases of skin disruption, oral medications may also be prescribed. On the natural remedy front, a soothing bath in which bleach or vinegar has been diluted can help decrease the skin bacteria that feed the

problem. For acne, daily application of vitamin A–based retinoid creams, gels, and lotions helps keep oil from filling hair follicles; antibacterial cream with salicylic acid also protects skin from breakouts.

Why CBD or Medical Cannabis Might Be the Answer

According to the National Eczema Association, the earliest medical advocate of cannabis for healing dermatitis may have been Dr. Henry Granger Piffard, who was one of the founders of American dermatology in the early 20th century. He wrote: "A pill of cannabis indica at bedtime has at my hands sometimes afforded relief to the intolerable itching of eczema."

Among several studies in the 21st century that have shown the antimicrobial, anti-inflammatory properties of cannabis, one in Germany, in 2006, demonstrated that cannabinoid-rich products soothe itching when applied to sites with eczema and other skin inflammations. In the case of psoriasis, CBD and other cannabinoids appear to inhibit the overproliferation of cells that cause plaque. Acne sufferers have also found that CBD lowers inflammation.

Not only has a 2018 issue of *Practical Dermatology* touted trials with cannabis that have relieved itching, ended mild atopic dermatitis, and shortened flare-ups, but a review of all recent studies on cannabis and skin conditions in a 2018 issue of *Dermatology Online* also found that cannabis products have been shown to be useful in treating acne, dermatitis, psoriasis, skin cancer, and much more. Both studies supported more in-depth investigations.

SUPPORTING RESEARCH

A 2019 article in the journal *Molecules* notes that studies over two decades have shown that skin tissue holds CB1 and CB2 receptors and their signaling is "deeply involved" in maintaining and regenerating skin and strengthening barriers that keep out infection—including dermatitis, acne, and cancers.

Research shows that CBD, in particular, interacts with CB2 receptors to calm inflammation and inhibit the over-proliferation of cells that cause the buildup of plaque. A 2018 issue of *Practical Dermatology* reported on at least two studies on mice in which THC interacted with CB1 receptors to suppress allergic contact dermatitis. It also cited a human study in which a cannabis medicinal got rid of mild dermatitis and prevented relapse in 80 percent of the participants.

In the case of acne, CBD has been found to deliver anti-acne activity by tamping down oil production from sebaceous glands and lowering inflammation. Compounds in cannabis that also help skin heal include the terpene limonene, which fights bacteria involved in acne infection, and the terpene linalool, which works against inflammation.

"*I hid my psoriasis under my makeup for four years. It didn't look nice, and I never wore short-sleeve tops because people would ask how I hurt myself. It looked like burns. It got worse with stress, and I have a stressful job, so I was always dealing with bad flare-ups. I noticed the difference using a [CBD] tincture within a month. It took three months to clear completely, but now I have normal skin. It really works.*"

—Dani, 26, Graduate Student

Integrative Tip >>>>>
While hemp seed oil does not contain any cannabinoids, it is a rich healer and has also been used on eczema with success. A 2018 report in the *International Journal of Molecular Sciences* noted the lubricating and healing benefits of plant oils for keeping the skin barrier strong against environmental invaders, as well as being antioxidant, anti-inflammatory, antimicrobial, wound healing, and anticarcinogenic.

30) Stress

Along with inflammation, stress may be one of the greatest general contributors to long-term body breakdown. Like inflammation, we all need some stress. It keeps us on our toes and alert to potentially harmful situations. But also like inflammation, too much stress over too long a period will begin to infiltrate the body in ways you've never imagined, triggering physical and

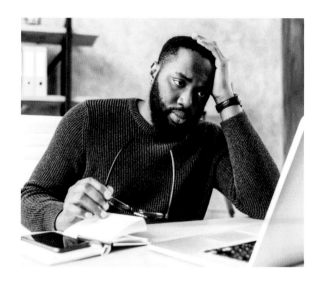

psychological illness and even early death. While many of us believe we cope with stress by working extra hours, shortening sleep to balance family time and relationships with work, missing meals—or eating junk food instead—in order to take on an extra task, or ending the day with a relaxing alcoholic drink or two, these Band-Aids® actually do very little to improve our general well-being, and over time, they can lead to anxiety, depression, memory loss, chronic pain, and even post-traumatic stress. Here's what happens: According to a 2016 NIH study on the interaction between stress and the ECS (endocannabinoid system), chronic stress decreases the production of both the ECS receptors in your body and the endocannabinoids that interact with them. The result? Your body's potential to fight inflammation and boost immune function is compromised. When your health is further compromised by loss of sleep, lack of exercise, and poor diet,

decline is inevitable. Any disorders that you may already have—including high blood pressure, indigestion, obesity, or obsessive-compulsive tendencies—become aggravated, and healthy operations, such as tissue repair, digestive function, detoxification, and coping, are derailed. Poor habits feed illness, which then feeds more poor habits. It's a hamster wheel, but you're not doomed to stay on it!

Current Remedies

Scientific research has shown that natural remedies, including walking outdoors, sniffing lavender, and listening to choral music, notably "Miserere" by Gregorio Allegri, calm stress. Alternatively, a range of medications may be prescribed. Sedatives and antidepressants are two options. Sedatives, which inhibit central nervous system activity to prompt relaxation, include a group called benzodiazepines, of which alprazolam (Xanax) and diazepam (Valium) are widely prescribed. Antidepressants, especially selective serotonin reuptake inhibitors (SSRIs), block the body's overly efficient uptake of serotonin, a chemical that prompts relaxation. Slowing uptake keeps serotonin in the system for a longer time to deliver calm and well-being. SSRIs include well-known brands like Prozac, Celexa®, and Paxil. Working closely with a physician is key to ensuring that pharmaceuticals like those don't counteract your existing drug regimen or become addictive.

Why CBD or Medical Cannabis Might Be the Answer

In her practice, cannabis expert Dr. Mary observes, "I typically hear people say that while taking cannabis, they not only feel like their sleep is improved but also that the stress that contributes to their difficulty with falling asleep or staying asleep is dramatically reduced. The stress reduction is the key to a good night's sleep." In 2018, the *Journal of Affective Disorders* published one of the first scientific studies to help people identify the most effective strains of cannabis—and the correct quantities to use—for treating stress and its associated ailments: anxiety and depression. Scientists deduced that smoking cannabis with varying levels of THC and CBD can enhance a patient's well-being and help reduce stress, anxiety, and depression in small, short-term doses. The study allowed patients to smoke various combinations of cannabis in the comfort of their own homes, instead of taking pills in a laboratory setting. The greatest relief from stress appeared to come with 10 or more puffs of cannabis that had both high-CBD and high-THC content. However, long-term use of cannabis at those elevated levels of CBD and THC appeared to have the opposite effect, exacerbating stress and related concerns. So a long-term answer may lie in adjusting and balancing strains.

SUPPORTING RESEARCH

According to a 2016 article in the journal *Neuropsychopharmacology*, "A growing body of work indicates that the endocannabinoid system (ECS) is an integral regulator of the stress response." Chronic stress has been shown to decrease endocannabinoid activity and tone, i.e., the well-balanced operation of the ECS. CBD and THC, along with certain other beneficial cannabis plant chemicals called terpenes, may help boost endocannabinoid function and prompt the release of the soothing natural chemicals serotonin and dopamine through the 5-HT1A receptor.

" You have to do your research before you start treatment. Cannabis strains and modes of administration are complicated, and there are a lot of products out there. You have to talk to your doctor. For me, it's a combination of a healthy diet, exercise, meditation, and taking the cannabis prescribed by my doctor. That's the combination that is making me feel better as a whole. "

—Angela, 62, RN

Integrative Tip >>>>>

About to take a test? Make a speech? Break bad news to someone you love? By making your breath the dominant focus, you'll lower your body's innate fight-or-flight response to fear and place negative thoughts on the back burner. First, choose a word that calms you. Then, sitting comfortably in a quiet place, close your eyes and breathe in slowly through your nose for 10 counts, allowing your chest and belly to rise and your abdomen to expand. Then breathe out slowly for 10 more counts, repeating the calming word. Continue this exercise for 10 minutes or longer.

31) Tics and Tourette Syndrome (TS)/ Stuttering

In the 2019 film *Motherless Brooklyn*, the protagonist, a detective played by actor Edward Norton, consistently stutters, opens his mouth, and shrugs his shoulders. He calls out, "I got threads in my head, I got threads in my head, I got threads in my head, man." Similar movements and "threads" are caused by Tourette syndrome (TS), a condition that affects more than 200,000 people across the United States.

Tourette syndrome is a neurological disorder. It was first documented in 1885 by groundbreaking French neurologist Dr. Georges Gilles as he worked with an elderly French noblewoman. Symptoms of the disorder include involuntary movements—motor tics, such as mouth opening, shoulder shrugging, head jerking, and eye blinking—as well as vocal tics that include the repetition of words or sounds, like *hmmm.* Boys experience the syndrome three to four times more often than girls. Usually, it appears in childhood between ages three and nine. Tics generally heighten in the teenage years and then may gradually improve with speech and medication therapy as a teen moves into adulthood.

Tics can be simple or complex, ranging from sniffing and grunting to touching objects, hopping, and barking. A person may compulsively repeat what someone else has said (echolalia); in some instances, the person may compulsively utter or repeat words that are inappropriate or obscene (coprolalia). Excitement and anxiety may provoke or worsen a tic, as can a tight collar or hearing someone else sniff or clear their throat. During sleep, symptoms may ease, but they never fully stop. Insomnia, anxiety, and depression may set in.

Studies show that TS is likely inherited, but researchers also believe that environmental factors, such as prenatal smoking by the mother and a mother's exposure to toxins while pregnant, may play a part. It is believed that the brain chemicals dopamine and serotonin play a role. The child of a Tourette's patient may not necessarily develop symptoms or, if they do, symptoms may be mild.

Genetic counseling may be recommended.

Current Remedies

Tourette syndrome is often misdiagnosed in the beginning as simple stuttering. Parents may invest in years of speech therapy, which can be helpful but doesn't address the heart of the problem. Once TS is diagnosed correctly, medications may not be fully effective and may be fraught with considerable side effects. Neuroleptics, drugs that depress nerve functions, i.e., tranquilizers, such as haloperidol and pimozide, may be used to treat psychotic and nonpsychotic disorders, such as suppressing tics.

But these medications can cause all kinds of problems, including dry mouth, blurred vision, muscle fatigue, cramping, and hazy cognitive function. It is not unusual for patients to gain upward of 50 pounds while ingesting such medications. Looking at the existing studies, there is room for new therapies—and they would be welcome. Researchers are working across disciplines in genetics, neuroimaging, neuropathology, and neurophysiology, as well as holding drug- and non-drug-based clinical trials to find out more.

Why CBD or Medical Cannabis Might Be the Answer

Patients with Tourette syndrome have found relief from their symptoms by utilizing synthetic THC and medical cannabis. Some case studies show a 70 percent reduction in tics and a 25 percent improvement in speech.

In a 2017 article published in the *International Journal of Molecular Sciences*, two cases involving German youths who had suffered from Tourette syndrome since childhood showed dramatic improvement with the administration of cannabis. One of the youths had suffered with stuttering, tics, and pronouncing the *hmmm* sound since the age of three. By the time he was eight years old, additional tics—stamping, blinking, kicking, and animal noises—made learning and socialization almost impossible. Throughout his adolescence, speech therapy and antipsychotic medications made little improvement, and by age

19 the patient was unable to hold a normal conversation; sometimes it took up to a minute for him to utter a single word. Insurance refused to cover the cost of synthetic THC, so the patient was started on medical cannabis using a vape. Eight months after the start of treatment, there was significant improvement: The patient experienced a 70 percent reduction in motor tics and was able to converse fluently in most situations. Even though the effects of THC were short, lasting only about 90 minutes, an ongoing sense of calm replaced the patient's anxiety and chronic stress.

In a particularly good study published in 2003 in the *Journal of Clinical Psychology,* 24 Tourette's patients filled out questionnaires and were followed by video, over a period of six weeks, as they were treated with THC-predominant cannabinoids. Researchers who came blind to the study—that is, with no previous knowledge of it—reviewed the videos and determined without bias whether the 24 patients had any reduction in vocal and motor tics. After just 10 days, there were considerable improvements—and those improvements continued. The videos offered other valuable data as well. Just 1 of the 24 patients left the study, an unusually low dropout rate, indicating that besides being well-tolerated, the cannabinoids likely had fewer significant side effects than other medications.

Another important takeaway to consider comes from a study published in the journal *Pharmacopsychiatry* in 2001, in which 12 Tourette's patients were given a single high dose of THC-predominant cannabinoids. Although some symptoms were controlled, others were not. Researchers scratched their heads. What we've concluded since then is that one dose of any medication can't determine outcome. A serious condition requires dosing several times over a period of four to six weeks to find the most effective dosing regimen. It's important to give yourself plenty of time for titration to adequately assess if the product is working.

SUPPORTING RESEARCH

While scientists do not know the cause of Tourette syndrome, research indicates that it is complex. Abnormalities in the brain's basal ganglia, frontal lobes, and cortex may be responsible, as well as the nerve circuitry that connects them. In addition, neurotransmitters, including dopamine and serotonin, do not appear to help the nerve cells communicate. Because research has shown that endocannabinoid system (ECS) receptors are also densely located in those parts of the brain, many experts believe that shoring up the ECS by ingesting cannabinoids may help ease symptoms. Ongoing, focused studies appear to support this belief. Because TS can provoke and be provoked by insomnia, stress, anxiety, and depression, cannabis may also be used to treat those symptoms. (See also "Anxiety," page 53; "Depression," page 70; "Insomnia," page 101; and "Stress," page 136.)

> **"** *I'm not a pothead. I don't care if you smoke. I've had Tourette's since I was a child. My stuttering isn't much better, even though I've been prescribed a cocktail of drugs my whole life. It is exhausting and frustrating to have Tourette's. The drugs have pretty negative side effects. Cannabis has helped with the movements at least, and that gives me hope.* **"**
>
> —Rennie, 30, Statistician

Integrative Tip > > > > >

Put on your mindset each morning just as you'd put on your clothes. Even with the most severe conditions of chronic disease, your thoughts and behaviors impact others. Make a decision each day about how you will "show up" in your life and how your actions and behaviors will impact others.

32) Weight Management

Fat is a beautiful thing. It defines us, giving us shape and vitality. And it is a lifesaver, padding us against surprise impacts that bring broken bones and internal injury. But too much fat—overweight—throws off our finely tuned body balance. The condition of being intensely overweight is called obesity and is defined as a chronic imbalance between energy intake and expenditure. That definition may make weight maintenance and control sound eminently simple: I'll just decrease energy intake or increase energy expenditure and excess weight will fall right off! Not true.

Despite years of intense research in the laboratory and clinic, researchers still find that the process of controlling weight gain and loss remains elusive. But they do know this: Added weight increases the risk of developing multiple chronic medical conditions, such as high blood pressure, diabetes, and high cholesterol. Overweight syndromes are associated with decreased quality of life and shortened life span and can increase the rate of depression in affected individuals. Obesity is associated with increased risk of several cancers—as high as 16 times greater in an obese person than in a person of healthy weight.

When we're out of balance, we may seek interventions that bring us back into balance quickly, rather than looking for an alternative that leads to long-term maintenance of homeostasis. The stress and anxiety of living in our current culture are monumental. It makes sense that if you are living on our planet today and reading this book, you are likely struggling with managing your stress and dealing with intermittent episodes of anxiety and depression. All that stress is throwing off your cortisol levels and depleting your feel-good neurotransmitters. So what do we do to feel better quickly? We eat! And it's creamy, sugar-rich, high–trans fat foods that bring on that quick fix, sadly—not fruits and veggies.

Our culture may not support a healthy lifestyle —but we are lucky to live at a time when there is more understanding than ever before about how to help your body naturally restore homeostasis with plant-based formulations. Restoring the tone of the ECS (endocannabinoid system) with CBD can lead to the balance that's missing in our current culture and provide the protection from unhealthy responses to stress that promote weight gain.

Current Treatments

Several prescription therapies have attempted to stimulate the metabolic pathways to aid weight loss. But most have had significant side effects, perhaps damaging the heart and, in the long run, actually slowing metabolism and causing weight to return. Multiple other interventions have focused on controlling caloric intake or increasing energy expenditure through diet and exercise: boot camps, calorie restriction, or diets that restrict certain foods, such as keto, paleo, and vegan, to name just a few. Many of these diets are meant to be used for short-term weight loss and may omit key nutrients over time.

Why CBD or Medical Cannabis Might Be the Answer

The magic ingredient may lie outside of diet and exercise. It may be possible to support healthy weight loss by stimulating the pleasure centers of the brain—not through eating or movement but by improving the tone of the endocannabinoid system through use of CBD and medical marijuana. Triggers for overeating, such as anxiety, depression, trauma, and stress, are often emotional. Because CBD and cannabis formulations can get to those roots, they can help stem the eating tide in a couple of different ways. One way, studies show, is by stimulating the ECS's CB1 receptors to increase a sense of reward similar to the one we experience when we eat. The other way is by interacting with the same receptors to decrease appetite. Find out why below.

SUPPORTING RESEARCH

The ECS helps to regulate appetite via the hypothalamus, which in turn modulates the reward functions in the brain that are associated with eating and other pleasurable pursuits, like hanging out with your family and friends and enjoying your favorite activities. The ECS can also support a healthy metabolism. Cannabinoid (CB) receptors CB1 and CB2 are present in every tissue and organ in the body, working to help you control inflammation and manage pain and stress. Within the brain and spinal cord, the ECS has multiple functions, but one function is to control energy balance.

Early research into the ECS concluded that blocking the CB1 receptor and limiting the stimulation of the system with cannabinoids decreased appetite and eating. This led to the development of the first CB1 receptor–blocker medication, which was introduced as a weight-loss drug in Europe in 2006. Unfortunately, depression and other psychiatric side effects occur when you block the reward pathways, and for those who took the receptor-blocker medication, not only was eating food less enjoyable but many other activities were also less

enjoyable, decreasing quality of life. The drug was taken off the market in 2008. Scientists then went back to the laboratory to find out exactly how to help people lose weight by working with the ECS.

Even though cannabis use has historically been associated with the munchies, it seems that only certain strains lead to—and only certain individuals experience—increased appetite when taking cannabis formulations. Generally speaking, individuals who use cannabinoid formulations maintain lower body weights over their lifetime, often maintaining the elusive "high school body weight" that is particularly healthy. This lower BMI (body mass index) is found in individuals with healthy ECS tone, which is often boosted by cannabinoid intake. Thus the toned ECS is linked to all the metabolic pluses achieved through regular use of cannabinoid formulations: decreased triglyceride levels, healthier cholesterol ratios, lower levels of insulin resistance, and better waist-to-hip ratios. Some might think that these indicators of a robust metabolism might simply be due to maintaining a lower BMI, but active studies are showing that regular cannabinoid use has a profoundly positive impact on healthy metabolism.

Exactly why stimulation of the ECS leads to weight control is still unclear, but researchers have come up with a number of ideas. The ECS works within the hypothalamus, improving pleasure and reward responses as described above, but it's also coupled with fat cells, signaling a stimulation of lipoprotein lipase, an enzyme that can change fat distribution and lower total fat cell count. This interaction can lead to weight loss and prevention of diet-induced obesity.

THC, the psychoactive portion of cannabis, is known to stimulate appetite and promote hunger, but other cannabinoids, such as CBD, may help to reduce appetite, control hunger, and decrease the total number of fat cells, promoting weight loss through the control of enzyme activity in the stored fats of the body. CBD may also decrease the anxiety many people feel when it comes to food and weight control, easing the struggle to control cravings.

Stimulation of the ECS may also result in weight control by changing the gut microbiome. Regular cannabinoid users not only have lower BMIs over their lifetimes but also seem to have healthy gut microbiome, which regulates growth of new fat cells as well as fat storage and fat metabolism. Cannabinoid formulations may help change levels and function of good bacteria, called Akkermansia muciniphila, which are involved in weight control and may promote weight loss.

Finally, improved ECS tone simply helps people feel better. A toned ECS prompts an increase in the release of serotonin, norepinephrine, and gabapentin in the nervous system. These feel-good neurotransmitters increase with food intake but also with intake of cannabinoids—without eating any food or doing any exercise or really doing anything else. Consuming cannabinoids helps to support a happier mood.

"Marijuana—it's the magic plant. There's nothing like it. I've lost 60 pounds in three years. It works better than anything else. I smoke one to three inhalations of marijuana before meals and then eat more vegetables and smoothies. Marijuana has cannabinoids in it, and cannabinoids do incredible things for bodies."

—**David, 53, Sales Executive**

Integrative Tip > > > > >

In one small study, people who started their meal with salad as the first course, ate 12 percent fewer calories. If dinner is usually 750 calories and a salad is added to the meal each night, a person can lose 9.4 pounds in one year.

Caroline Hartridge, DO

Caroline Hartridge, a doctor of osteopathic medicine, is licensed as a general practitioner in New York and Georgia. Dr. Hartridge works with a wide range of chronic and acute conditions, helping address them with osteopathic manipulative medicine and plant-based nutrition counseling. She is also a New York State medical marijuana–referring physician. In addition to being a physician, Dr. Hartridge has developed a CBD-isolate product line and serves on the board of several nonprofits in the US and Puerto Rico.

33) Women's Health

"I am woman, hear me roar!" That line, from Helen Reddy's classic "I Am Woman," is inspiring. It's also true—we roar when we are angry, righteous, and, yes—when we're in menstrual pain.

While a woman's monthly cycle sets the stage for her wondrous ability to conceive and bear children, premenstrual syndrome (PMS) and the pain that accompanies each menstrual cycle are generally dreaded. According to the US Department of Health and Human Services Office on Women's Health, more than 90 percent of women experience PMS. As hormones fluctuate in preparation for the uterus to start sloughing off the lining it has built up over the last 28 days, a women may experience abdominal bloating, cramping, headaches, fuzzy brain, breast tenderness, moodiness, carbohydrate cravings, and anxiety—sometimes debilitatingly so.

Many women also suffer from endometriosis, a condition in which tissue that normally lines the uterus grows outside it—on the ovaries, fallopian tubes, or on the intestines. Along with the uterus, these other nests of endometrial tissue in the abdomen also go through monthly cycles, leading to pain and disability. Even gut function is affected. Outside of menstruation, pain can occur during intercourse or urination, and the condition may be the precursor to ovarian cancer.

Endometriosis can also affect fertility, but there are other causes, too, such as reduced hormone levels. A woman may not have appropriate estrogen and progesterone release to help her uterus prepare for and maintain a pregnancy. Endometriosis and hormone release issues are among the reasons why 10–18 percent of couples have trouble conceiving and successfully bringing a baby to term. The good news, according to Mayo Clinic, is that about 95 percent of couples do successfully conceive after two years of trying—with or without treatment.

As childbearing years draw to a close and the ovaries retire, menopause sets in. Shutdown of the monthly cycle brings relief, but other bodily discomforts step in: hot flashes, night sweats, vaginal dryness, lack of concentration, insomnia, slowing metabolism with weight gain, and thinning nails, hair, and bones. While going through the process is no fun, it is also freeing to be on the other side. Your brain regains its sharpness, sex is pregnancy-worry-free, and you've established who you are. Your wisdom and womanhood bring a new kind of roar: celebration.

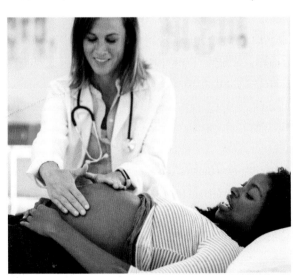

Current Treatments

Help for PMS may come in the form of aspirin, ibuprofen, or heat application. A doctor may prescribe antidepressants and antianxiety medicine for emotional swings or diuretics for bloating. We can, of course, do all kinds of things medically to help women have a menstrual cycle less frequently, such as hormonal birth control therapies that limit the frequency of menstruation or stop menstruation altogether. These hormonal therapies can make a remarkable difference for people who are suffering with menstrual pain, but they're not for everyone. Some women worry about increased risk of blood clots or breast cancer while on hormone therapy.

Endometriosis requires more serious attention. If the condition is exceptionally painful and inhibiting fertility, a physician may recommend surgery.

In the case of menopause, conventional treatment has long focused on hormone replacement therapy (HRT)—the combined use of estrogen and progesterone to replace the estrogen your body stops making during menopause. But women at risk for breast cancer can't use any kind of HRT. Alternative prescription medications can help, as well as lifestyle changes for insomnia-prompting night sweats—such as wearing cotton nightclothes and using a mattress pad without a rubber backing.

For women's health in general, diet is key: Eating anti-inflammatory fruits and vegetables—and not giving in to carb and sugar cravings—will help control bloating and mood swings. Some research has been done on hemp seed oil; the omega-3 and omega-6 fatty acids in the oil have been found to help stabilize fluctuating blood sugar levels that may contribute to PMS. And then there is body- and soul-lifting exercise: For women at all stages of life, picking up the pace can help ease menstrual cramps, clear and sharpen a fuzzy brain, induce sleep, and lift mood.

Why CBD or Medical Cannabis Might Be the Answer

Can cannabinoids help with pain related to menstrual periods? Research says yes. In one study, mice that were given THC were found to have reductions in endometrial activity. They had less pain and less dysfunction related to pain, in addition to better mood. The mice also benefited from improved memory with cannabis administration, after experiencing memory difficulties related to episodes of painful endometriosis.

An Australian study published by *Journal of Obstetrics and Gynaecology Canada* in 2020 asked several hundred women who suffered with endometriosis to describe the alternative and complementary therapies they were using, apart from their doctors' interventions, to try to get their endometrial pain under control. Out of this group, 13 percent reported that they were regularly using cannabis to control their endometrial pain. They might be onto something.

Because of a cannabis prohibition in Australia, there may actually be even more women using cannabis regularly who aren't informing researchers. Out of the 13 percent who said cannabis helped, 56 percent reported significant improvement in their endometrial symptoms. So the human findings would appear to support the mouse findings: In the mouse model we saw evidence of decreasing behavior that indicated pain, decreased anxiety, and improved memory; in humans we saw that women decreased their pharmaceutical pain management by half and also reported improved sleep and less nausea and vomiting.

So, for women with endometriosis, there is, potentially, a great opportunity to offer them more relief with cannabinoids. There are other benefits, too: For patients who are dealing with very painful or heavy menstrual cycles, cannabinoids can help.

SUPPORTING RESEARCH

It makes sense that cannabis decreases cramps and pain because CB1 receptors are present in the lining of the uterus and their stimulation by cannabinoids can help reduce local inflammation and pain. Also, by working with CB1 receptors located throughout the central nervous system, cannabinoids can help decrease pain pathway responses in the spine and brain. Through interaction with receptors in the brain cannabinoids may also help get rid of brain fog.

In addition, cannabinoids can help make menstrual sloughing less intense. It turns out that for women who use cannabinoids, there is an actual reduction in gonadotropin-releasing hormone, GnRH, which is secreted by the pituitary gland. GnRH is responsible for the subsequent secretion of progesterone and estrogen, important hormones that help regulate the menstrual cycle. Secretion of less estrogen and progesterone effectively reduces the amount of endometrial tissue that needs to be sloughed off at the end of the cycle. Cannabis also helps to decrease endometrial tissue by stimulating CB1 receptors in the uterus. If you're having a lot of painful periods, the use of cannabis to reduce GnRH and, subsequently, estrogen and progesterone—and also stimulate the CB receptors in the uterus—may be exactly what you need to have a better life.

However, it's important to recognize that the impact of cannabinoids on the endometrium is both positive and negative. While cannabinoids may help relieve endometriosis pain and heavy menses, they may negatively impact female fertility. That's because, in making menstruation less painful and heavy, they also lower estrogen and progesterone levels. For infertile women, appropriate estrogen and progesterone release is necessary, and reduced hormone levels through cannabis use may further compromise the ability to conceive. If you're experiencing a fertility issue, hold off on cannabinoid use. It may be limiting the ability of the uterine lining to build and grow to the thickness required for an egg to implant.

In a Canadian study reported in *BC Medical Journal* in 2019, it was found that about 13 percent of almost 300 infertile women had reported using cannabinoid formulations in the past year; that's concerning to scientists who study the way cannabinoids work in the brain and throughout the body.

In the case of menopause, the ECS would appear to have lost tone and become endocannabinoid-deficient. Cannabinoids may help restore balance to the ECS. Cannabis in the form of THC has been reported to ease hot flashes, and CBD has been found to help alleviate the depression and bone loss that can accompany this change of life (see "Depression," page 71).

Research shows that cannabinoid interactions with the ECS can help ease the anxiety, stress, and insomnia that accompany each of the aforementioned conditions. (See "Anxiety," page 53; "Stress," page 136; and "Insomnia," page 101.)

" The pain was so intense, like a throbbing or a burning cramp in my pelvis. The pain would shoot into my lower back and my thighs. For the first two days, I couldn't go to school or work. I'd be crying from the pain. I felt angry and frustrated because of my circumstances. I felt like a prisoner in my body. My primary care doctor told me the pain was normal and part of being a woman. I would treat it with a heating pad or a hot bath, but exercise or even ordinary movements were impossible. I saw the effects of cannabis in just two months, and my cycle became more normal. If I forget to take it, the pain comes back just like before. It's a huge relief to have my life back. I can shop and work and do all kinds of normal things again. "

—Meeghan, 24, Flight Attendant

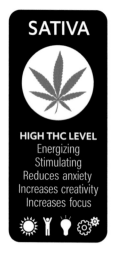
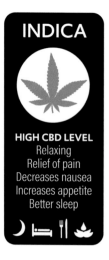
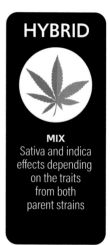

SATIVA

HIGH THC LEVEL
Energizing
Stimulating
Reduces anxiety
Increases creativity
Increases focus

INDICA

HIGH CBD LEVEL
Relaxing
Relief of pain
Decreases nausea
Increases appetite
Better sleep

HYBRID

MIX
Sativa and indica
effects depending
on the traits
from both
parent strains

Dr. Anna Cabeca

When Dr. Anna Cabeca was diagnosed with early menopause at age 38, she was devastated. Undaunted, this triple board–certified, Emory University–trained physician and hormone expert then set out on a personal wellness journey to reverse the side effects of menopause. At age 41, Cabeca delivered a healthy baby girl and began counseling others, ultimately changing the lives of thousands of women around the globe. Her book *The Hormone Fix* and her life-changing products and programs have helped women of all ages become their best selves again. Her all-natural products include the alkaline superfoods drink Mighty Maca® Plus and Julva®, a rejuvenating vulvar cream. In 2018, Dr. Cabeca was named "Innovator of the Year" by Mindshare Collaborative, the premier community for health and wellness influencers and entrepreneurs.

Integrative Tip > > > > >

Get seven to eight hours of sleep a night. Depriving your body of sleep adversely affects nervous system function, hormone release, and inflammatory chemicals that increase hunger, decrease satiety, and favor fat buildup. Studies have linked chronic insomnia to night-shift work, jet lag, and eating late.

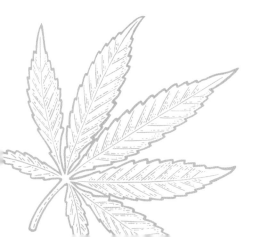

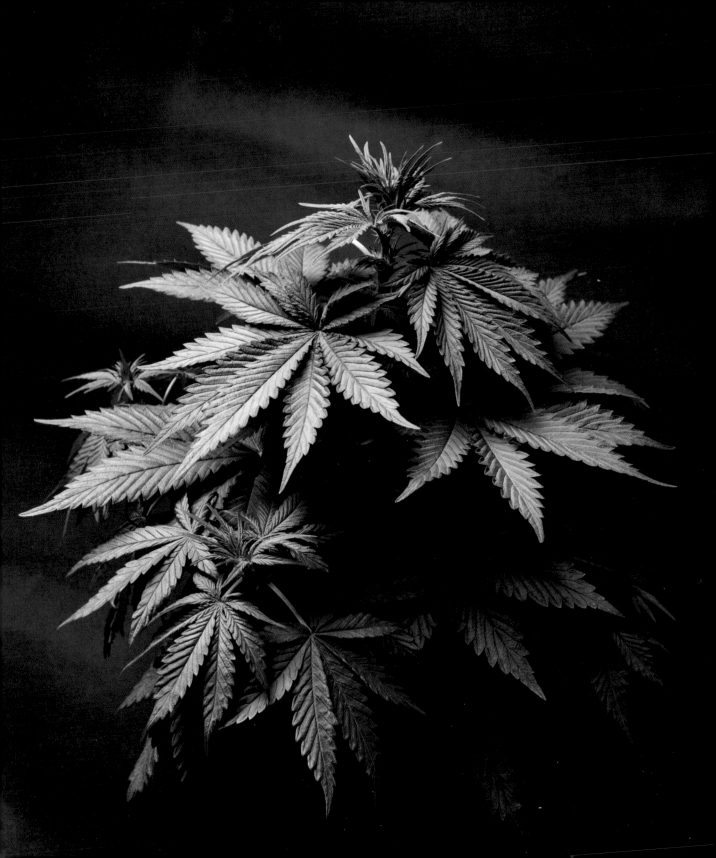

< Glossary >

amygdala   Almond-shaped part of the brain that plays a major role in emotion, behavior, and processing fear.

analgesic   Pain relieving.

anandamide   Often called the "bliss molecule," an endocannabinoid that has been found to help ease pain and depression.

antigen   A toxin or other harmful substance that triggers an immune response in the body.

anti-inflammatory
A substance that acts against chemicals that cause inflamed tissue, whether in arthritic joints or from insect stings and poison ivy.

antioxidant   A substance that prevents harmful molecules from oxidizing, a process of breaking down cells that contributes to cancer, arthritis, and other diseases.

autoimmune disease
A disease prompted by the immune system mistakenly attacking healthy body tissue.

basal ganglia   A deep part of the brain responsible for motor control and learning, executive function, behavior, and emotion.

blue zones   Areas around the world where people traditionally practice integrated health and live full and long lives.

bradykinesia   Slowness of movement

broad spectrum   A term referring to cannabis products that include CBD and other phytocannabinoids and nutrients from the cannabis plant but no THC.

< 151 >

cannabidiol   (also called CBD) A phytocannabinoid that populates the cannabis plant and has healing properties without the "high" that is triggered by other phytocannabinoids, such as THC (see "THC"). Research shows it is the most abundant of the phytocannabinoids.

cannabinoid formulation

A product containing the cannabinoids THC and CBD, such as oral drops, edibles, sprays, patches, or oils for vaporizing cartridges.

cannabinoids   A family of healing chemical compounds produced naturally in the body as well as in hemp and cannabis plants. They interact with the endocannabinoid system to help the body maintain homeostasis. In the body, they're called *endocannabinoids*; in plants, they're called *phytocannabinoids*. Some cannabis phytocannabinoids produce a high.

cannabinol   A mildly psychoactive by-product of degradation often found in improperly cared-for or aged cannabis.

cannabis   The plant umbrella name that includes CBD-rich hemp and THC-rich marijuana.

cardiomyopathy   Sometimes triggered by diabetes, this disease turns the heart muscle rigid and makes it unable to pump blood efficiently to the rest of the body.

CBD   See "Cannabidiol."

coprolalia   Often observed in Tourette syndrome, the tendency to compulsively utter or repeat words that are inappropriate or obscene.

cytokines   Proteins released by the immune system to fight a body stressor such as infection. The release of too many at once, called a cytokine storm, causes a harmful, inflammatory reaction.

demyelination   Damage to the protective covering—the myelin sheath—that surrounds nerve fibers.

dopaminergic drugs

These address low levels of dopamine due to impairment of neurons in the deep part of the brain, called the substantia nigra, where dopamine is produced.

dyskinesia   Involuntary, erratic, writhing movements of the face, arms, legs, or trunk, often a side effect of Parkinson's medication.

echolalia Often observed in Tourette syndrome, the tendency to compulsively utter or repeat someone else's words.

ECS See "Endocannabinoid System."

endocannabinoid A cannabinoid, a healing chemical compound that is naturally produced by the body. In plants, a similar compound is called a phytocannabinoid.

endocannabinoid system (ECS)

  A bodily system that helps maintain homeostasis, or balance, in body operations, such as inflammation control and healthy brain, nerve, circulation, and immune function, among other benefits.

endocannabinoid

  TONE The health of the endocannabinoid system. Optimal endocannabinoid tone means that all systems are humming along, working together harmoniously, and supporting a balanced, healthy body.

entourage effect

  What happens when you use products made with all the cannabis plant constituents; this has a more powerful healing effect than using products that isolate a cannabinoid such as THC or CBD. The more than 100 other cannabinoids in cannabis support one another to increase their individual power. This yields a richer, more lasting healing effect.

executive function

  The ability to perform a series of cognitive tasks to problem-solve effectively.

flavonoids A diverse group of phytonutrients (plant nutrients) that give fruits and vegetables their vivid colors. Flavonoids are antioxidant and packed with healing powers.

free radicals Unstable atoms with unpaired electrons, generated by the body, when it is exposed to pollutants and disease. To stabilize themselves, free radicals steal electrons from other molecules, causing a chain reaction of electron raiding that promotes oxidative stress, or cell damage and chronic illness.

full spectrum A term referring to a cannabis product that contains many phytocannabinoids and other nutrients, with both CBD and trace amounts of THC (under 0.3 percent).

HDL	High-density lipoproteins, which carry cholesterol from parts of the body to be disposed of by the liver. Often called "good cholesterol."
hemp	Also called industrial hemp, this is the umbrella family name for cannabis, and marijuana (*Cannabis sativa*) is the species. The two subspecies of cannabis are hemp (*Cannabis sativa sativa*) and recreational marijuana (*Cannabis sativa indica*).
hemp CBD product	A product made from the hemp plant that contains more healing CBD than THC. Legal hemp CBD products contain less than 0.3 percent THC. Such products can be purchased as alcohol- or oil-based tinctures, oils, isolate powders, foods, and topical salves and balms.
hippocampus	The part of the brain that plays a major role in learning and memory.
homeostasis	The balance of all bodily systems for optimal function and health.
hormonal	Referring to hormones or endocrine system function.
hybrid	A cross between Indica and Sativa, a hybrid strain of cannabis can help medical marijuana patients find the right product for their individual needs.
integrated health	The practice of keeping the whole body healthy through six pillars: sleep, stress management, balanced diet, exercise, spirituality, socialization.
isolate	A product that is refined into a powder—a single-focus cannabinoid—"isolating" it from any oils, fatty acids, or other plant components that may contribute to a full-healing entourage effect. An isolate can more quickly address certain conditions.
LDL	Low-density lipoproteins, which remain in the body and build up in the arteries, eventually causing heart attack or stroke. Often called "bad cholesterol."
macrophages	White blood cells that fight infection.
metabolite	The end product present in your body after it breaks down a substance; for instance, after THC metabolizes in the body, it is stored in body fat as the metabolite THC-COOH. Drug tests look for this metabolite to indicate THC usage.

myelin sheath   The protective covering around nerve fibers that supports the efficient transmission of electrical pulses along nerve cells.

neurotransmitter   Chemicals made by nerve cells that transmit messages from that nerve cell to another nerve cell, or a muscle or gland cell.

omega-3 fatty acids

Essential fats (ingested through diet) that support healthy heart, brain, and metabolic function.

omega-6 fatty acids

Essential fats (ingested through diet) that deliver energy to the body and aid in healthy inflammatory response to injury and disease. However, too many omega-6s, through the Western diet of polyunsaturated fats and fast foods, can trigger unhealthy inflammation that leads to disease.

oxidation   Cell damage caused by free radicals. It's the same process that rusts a car or turns an apple brown.

phytocannabinoids

Some 100 kinds of healing chemical compounds (among other plant nutrients) likely produced exclusively in the cannabis plant. To date, cannabidiol (CBD) is known to be the most abundant kind of phytocannabinoid.

plant nutrients or phytonutrients

Chemicals produced by plants to protect the plant from germs, fungus, and other threats, and which are transferred to us through plant foods, promoting efficient body function. Examples: cannabinoids, carotenoids, ellagic acid, flavonoids, and terpenes.

plaques   Raised red patches that occur in cases of dermatitis. Plaques may also be the result of cholesterol deposition in blood vessels that calcify over time and cause restricted blood flow and vascular disease.

REM   Rapid eye movement sleep, one of four sleep stages, is the one during which you usually dream. Memory consolidation takes place during this time, but also during non-REM sleep.

resin   Sticky, dewlike drops covering the cannabis plant, from which healing components are extracted to make medicine; hemp is not as rich in resin as is marijuana.

SPF   Sun protection factor, found on sunscreen products, specifically indicating protection against the sun's harmful ultraviolet rays that cause sunburn.

substantia nigra   Part of the basal ganglia in the deep brain, governing movement and reward functions.

synovial fluid   Thick fluid that cushions the joints of arms, legs, and fingers.

terpenes   Including limonene and pinene, terpenes are responsible for the aroma of cannabis and for fighting unhealthy inflammation and cell deterioration. They are also natural bug repellents, especially limonene.

tetrahydrocannabinal
                       (also called THC) A phytocannabinoid found in hemp and marijuana plants that both heals and, in large concentration, causes a "high" (psychoactivity).

THC   See "Tetrahydrocannabinol."

tincture   A delivery system for cannabis. Plant parts are soaked in ethanol (alcohol) to extract the active healing ingredients. Final products are either a straight alcohol tincture or one that has been diluted with oil (an oil-based alcohol tincture) or glycerin (a glycerin-based alcohol tincture) for less potent delivery.

titration   The process of starting at a low medicine dosage and gradually building up to determine its optimal healing effect on the body.

trichomes   Hairlike protrusions on the cannabis plant that contain resin. Called the "resin glands," they produce concentrated cannabinoids and terpenes.

tumor necrosis factor (TNF)
                       A highly inflammatory protein, often overproduced in rheumatoid arthritis patients.

< Selected Bibliography >

Abo-Elnazar, S., et al. "Th17/Treg Imbalance in Opioids and Cannabinoids Addiction: Relationship to NF-kB Activation in CD4+ T Cells." *Egyptian Journal of Immunology* (2014). https://pubmed.ncbi.nlm.nih.gov/25812351/.

Ahmed, Waseem. "Therapeutic Use of Cannabis in Inflammatory Bowel Disease." *Gasteroenterology and Hepatology* (2016). https://www.ncbi.nlm.nih.gov/pmc/articles/PMC5193087/.

Al-Ghezi, Zinah Zamil, et al. "Combination of Cannabinoids, Δ9-Tetrahydrocannabinol and Cannabidiol, Ameliorates Experimental Multiple Sclerosis by Suppressing Neuroinflammation through Regulation of miRNA-Mediated Signaling Pathways." *Frontiers of Immunology* (2019). https://www.ncbi.nlm.nih.gov/pmc/articles/PMC6712515/.

Allegretti, Ravikoff, et al. "Marijuana Use Patterns among Patients with Inflammatory Bowel Disease." *Inflammatory Bowel Disease* (2013). https://pubmed.ncbi.nlm.nih.gov/24185313/.

Amtmann, Dagmar. "Survey of Cannabis Use in Patients with Amyotrophic Lateral Sclerosis." *American Journal of Hospice and Palliative Care* (2004). https://www.ncbi.nlm.nih.gov/pubmed/15055508.

Andre, C., et al., "Cannabis Sativa: The Plant of One Thousand Molecules." *Frontiers in Plant Science* (2016). https://www.ncbi.nlm.nih.gov/pmc/articles/PMC4740396.

Andreae, Michael H., et al. Inhaled Cannabis for Chronic Neuropathic Pain: A Meta-analysis of Individual Patient Data." *Journal of Pain* (2015). https://www.ncbi.nlm.nih.gov/pubmed/26362106.

Arjmand, Shokouh, et al. "Bipolar Disorder and the Endocannabinoid System," *Acta Neuropsychiatrica* (2019). https://www.ncbi.nlm.nih.gov/pubmed/31159897.

Artigas, Maria Soler, et al. "Attention-Deficit/Hyperactivity Disorder and Lifetime Cannabis Use: Genetic Overlap and Causality." *Molecular Psychiatry* (2020). https://www.ncbi.nlm.nih.gov/pubmed/30610198.

Backes, Michael, with J. McCue, MD, eds. *Cannabis Pharmacy: The Practical Guide to Medical Marijuana*. New York: Black Dog & Leventhal Publishers, 2014.

< 157 >

Barchel, Dana, et al. "Oral Cannabidiol Use in Children with Autism Spectrum Disorder to Treat Related Symptoms and Co-morbidities." *Frontiers in Pharmacology* (2018). https://www.ncbi.nlm.nih.gov/pmc/articles/PMC6333745/.

Bar-Sela, G., et al. "The Medical Necessity for Medicinal Cannabis: Prospective Observational Study Evaluating the Treatment in Cancer Patients on Supportive or Palliative Care." *Evidence-Based Complementary Alternative Medicine* (2017). https://www.ncbi.nlm.nih.gov/pubmed/23956774.

Bassi, Mario Stampanoni. "Exploiting the Multifaceted Effects of Cannabinoids on Mood to Boost Their Therapeutic Use against Anxiety and Depression." *Frontiers in Molecular Neuroscience* (2018). https://www.ncbi.nlm.nih.gov/pmc/articles/PMC6256035/.

Bitencourt, R., and R. Takahashi. "Cannabidiol as a Therapeutic Alternative for Post-Traumatic Stress Disorder." *Frontiers in Neuroscience* (2018). https://www.ncbi.nlm.nih.gov/pmc/articles/PMC6066583/.

Booth, Martin. *Cannabis: A History.* New York: Picador, 2005.

Booz, G. W. "Cannabidiol as an Emergent Therapeutic Strategy for Lessening the Impact of Oxidative Stress." *Free Radical Biology & Medicine* (2011).

https://www.ncbi.nlm.nih.gov/pubmed/21238581.

Bransfield, Robert C. "Neuropsychiatric Lyme Borreliosis: An Overview with a Focus on a Specialty Psychiatrist's Clinical Practice." *Healthcare* (2018). https://www.ncbi.nlm.nih.gov/pmc/articles/PMC6165408/.

Bridgeman, M., et al. "Medicinal Cannabis: History, Pharmacology, and Implications for the Acute Care Setting." *Pharmacy and Therapeutics* (2017). https://www.ncbi.nlm.nih.gov/pmc/articles/PMC5312634/.

Brownell Grogan, Barbara. *CBD Handbook: Recipes for Natural Living.* New York: Sterling, 2020.

Cameron, Colin. "Use of a Synthetic Cannabinoid in a Correctional Population for Posttraumatic Stress Disorder–Related Insomnia and Nightmares, Chronic Pain, Harm Reduction, and Other Indications." *Journal of Clinical Psychopharmacology* (2014). https://www.ncbi.nlm.nih.gov/pmc/articles/PMC4165471/.

Cameron, Michelle, et al. "Effects of Cannabis on Cognitive Function in Patients with Multiple Sclerosis." *Neurology* (2011). https://www.ncbi.nlm.nih.gov/pmc/articles/PMC3068013/.

Carter, Gregory T. "Cannabis and Amyotrophic Lateral Sclerosis: Hypothetical and Practical Applications, and a Call for Clinical Trials." *American Journal of Hospice and Palliative Care* (2010). https://www.ncbi.nlm.nih.gov/pubmed/20439484.

Chagas, Marcos Hortes, et al. "Effects of Cannabidiol in the Treatment of Patients with Parkinson's Disease: An Exploratory Double-Blind Trial." *Journal of Psychopharmacology,* (2014). https://www.ncbi.nlm.nih.gov/pubmed/25237116.

Clifton, Mary, MD. CBD & Cannabis Library. https://cbdandcannabisinfo.com/.

Clifton, Mary, MD, and Tom O'Brien. *The Grass is Greener: Medial Marijuana, THC, and CBD Oil: Reversing Chronic Pain, Inflammation, and Disease.* New York: Book Baby, 2019.

Corroon, J., and J. A. Phillips. "A Cross-Sectional Study of Cannabidiol Users." *Cannabis and Cannabinoid Research* (2018). https://www.ncbi.nlm.nih.gov/pubmed/30014038.

Crippa, Jose Alexandre, et al. "Neural Basis of Anxiolytic Effects of Cannabidiol (CBD) in Generalized Social Anxiety Disorder: A Preliminary Report." *Journal of Psychopharmacology* (2011). https://www.ncbi.nlm.nih.gov/pubmed/20829306.

Cuttler, Carrie, et al. "Short- and Long-Term Effects of Cannabis on Headache and Migraine." *Journal of Pain* (2019). https://www.sciencedaily.com/releases/2019/11/191125100353.htm.

Dai, Hongying, and Kimber P. Richter. "A National Survey of Marijuana Use among US Adults with Medical Conditions, 2016–2017." *JAMA Network* (2019). https://jamanetwork.com/journals/jamanetworkopen/fullarticle/2751558.

Darkovska-Serafimoskva, M., et al. "Pharmacotherapeutic Considerations for Use of Cannabinoids to Relieve Pain in Patients with Malignant Diseases." *Journal of Pain Research* (2018). https://www.ncbi.nlm.nih.gov/pmc/articles/PMC5922297/.

Dmietrieva, N. "Endocannabinoid Involvement in Endometriosis." *Pain* (2010). https://www.ncbi.nlm.nih.gov/pubmed/20833475.

Dzierzanowski, Tomasz. "Prospects for the Use of Cannabinoids in Oncology and Palliative Care Practice: A Review of the Evidence." *Cancers* (2019) https://www.ncbi.nlm.nih.gov/pmc/articles/PMC6406915/.

Eagleston, Lauren R. M., et al. "Cannabinoids in Dermatology: A Scoping Review." *Dermatology Online* (2018). https://www.ncbi.nlm.nih.gov/pubmed/30142706.

Facci, L. et al. "Mast Cells Express a Peripheral Cannabinoid Receptor with Differential Sensitivity to Anandamide and Palmitoylethanolamide." *Proceedings of the National Academies of Science* (1995) https://www.ncbi.nlm.nih.gov/pmc/articles/PMC42169/.

Finseth, Taylor Andrew. "Self-Reported Efficacy of Cannabis and Other Complementary Medicine Modalities by Parkinson's Disease Patients in Colorado." *Evidence-Based Complementary Alternative Medicine* (2015). https://www.ncbi.nlm.nih.gov/pubmed/25821504.

Gladstar, Rosemary. *Rosemary Gladstar's Herbal Recipes for Vibrant Health: 175 Teas, Tonics, Oils, Salves, Tinctures, and Other Natural Remedies for the Entire Family.* North Adams, MA: Storey Publishing, 2008.

Grill, M., et al., "Medical Cannabis and Cannabinoids: An Option for the Treatment of Inflammatory Bowel Disease and Cancer of the Colon?" *Medical Cannabis and Cannabinoids* (2018). https://www.karger.com/Article/FullText/489036.

Grill, M. et al. "Cellular Localization and Regulation of Receptors and Enzymes of the Endocannabinoid System in Intestinal and Systemic Inflammation." *Histochemistry and Cell Biology* (2019). https://www.ncbi.nlm.nih.gov/pubmed/30196316.

Gruber, Staci. "The Grass Might Be Greener: Medical Marijuana Patients Exhibit Altered Brain Activity and Improved Executive Function after 3 Months of Treatment." *Frontiers of Pharmacology.* (2017). https://www.ncbi.nlm.nih.gov/pmc/articles/PMC5776082/.

Habib, G., and S. Artul. "Medical Cannabis for the Treatment of Fibromyalgia." *Journal of Clinical Rheumatology* (2018). https://www.ncbi.nlm.nih.gov/pubmed/29461346.

Hammell, D. C., et al. "Transdermal Cannabidiol Reduces Inflammation and Pain-Related Behaviors in a Rat Model of Arthritis." *European Journal of Pain* (2015). https://www.ncbi.nlm.nih.gov/pubmed/26517407.

Hausman-Kedem, Moran, et al. "Efficacy of CBD-Enriched Medical Cannabis for Treatment of Refractory Epilepsy in Children and Adolescents: An Observational, Longitudinal Study." *Brain & Development* (2018). https://www.ncbi.nlm.nih.gov/pubmed/29674131.

Herd, Yasmin, et al. "Early Phase in the Development of Cannabidiol as a Treatment for Addiction: Opioid Relapse Takes Initial Center Stage." *Neurotherapeutics* (2015). https://pubmed.ncbi.nlm.nih.gov/26269227/.

Hildebrand, Andrea, et al. "Cannabis Use for Symptom Relief in Multiple Sclerosis: A Cross-Sectional Survey of Webinar Attendees in the U.S. and Canada." *Multiple Sclerosis* (2019). https://www.msard-journal.com/article/S2211-0348(19)30837-5/abstract.

Holland, Julie, ed. *The Pot Book: A Complete Guide to Cannabis, Its Role in Medicine, Politics, Science, and Culture.* Rochester, VT: Park Street Press, 2010.

Huppli, A. M. M. "Medical Cannabis for Adult Attention Deficit Hyperactivity Disorder." *Medical Cannabis and Cannabinoids* (2018). https://www.karger.com/Article/Fulltext/495307.

Jackson, N. J., et al. "Impact of Adolescent Marijuana Use on Intelligence." *Proceedings of the National Academy of Sciences of the United States of America* (2017). https://pubmed.ncbi.nlm.nih.gov/26787878/.

Jakubovski, Ewgeni, and Kirsten Muller-Val. "Speechlessness in Gilles de la Tourette Syndrome: Cannabis-Based Medicines Improve Severe Vocal Blocking Tics in Two Patients." *International Journal of Molecular Sciences* (2017). https://www.ncbi.nlm.nih.gov/pubmed/28796166.

Jatoi A., et al. "Does Megestrol Acetate Down-Regulate Interleukin-6 in Patients with Cancer-Associated Anorexia and Weight Loss?" *Supportive Care in Cancer* (2002). https://pubmed.ncbi.nlm.nih.gov/11777191/.

Keen, Larry II, et al. "Differential Effects of Self-Reported Lifetime Marijuana Use on Interleukin-1 Alpha and Tumor Necrosis Factor in African American Adults." *Journal of Behavioral Medicine* (2015). https://www.ncbi.nlm.nih.gov/pmc/articles/PMC4425573/.

Kindred, John H. "Cannabis Use in People with Parkinson's Disease and Multiple Sclerosis: A Web-Based Investigation." *Complementary Therapies in Medicine* (2017). https://pubmed.ncbi.nlm.nih.gov/28735833/.

Klein, T. W. "Cannabinoid-Based Drugs As Anti-Inflammatory Therapeutics." *Nature Reviews—Immunology* (2005). https://pubmed.ncbi.nlm.nih.gov/15864274/.

Koubeissi, Mohamad. "Anticonvulsant Effects of Cannabidiol in Dravet Syndrome." *Epilepsy Currents* (2017). https://www.ncbi.nlm.nih.gov/pmc/articles/PMC5716495/.

Laegeforen, Tidsskr Nor. "Use of Benzodiazepines and Cannabis in Young Adults." *Pubmed* (2010). https://pubmed.ncbi.nlm.nih.gov/20453954/.

Lavie-Ajayi, Maya, and Pesach Schvartzman. "Restored Self: A Phenomenological Study of Pain Relief by Cannabis." *Pain Medicine* (2019). https://www.ncbi.nlm.nih.gov/pubmed/30215782.

Lee, Martin. "From Clone to Concentrate: How CBD Oil Is Made." *Project CBD* (2017). https://www.projectcbd.org/about/herbal-medicine/cloneconcentrate-how-cbd-oil-made.

———. "Interview with Dr. Ethan Russo: CBD, the Entourage Effect, and the Microbiome" *Project CBD* (2019). https://www.projectcbd.org/dr-ethan-russo-cbd-entourage-effect-and-microbiome.

———. *Smoke Signals: A Social History of Marijuana—Medical, Recreational, and Scientific.* New York: Scribner, 2012.

Leinow, Leonard, and Juliana Birnbaum. Foreword by Michael H. Moskowitz, MD. *CBD: A Patient's Guide to Medicinal Cannabis, Healing without the High.* Berkeley, CA: North Atlantic Books, 2017.

Leweke, F. M. "Cannabidiol Enhances Anandamide Signaling and Alleviates Psychotic Symptoms of Schizophrenia." *Translational Psychiatry* (2012). https://www.ncbi.nlm.nih.gov/pmc/articles/PMC3316151/.

Lidicker, Gretchen. *CBD Oil Everyday Secrets: A Lifestyle Guide to Hemp-Derived Health and Wellness*. New York: The Countryman Press/W. W. Norton, 2018.

Lloyd, Shawnta L., and Catherine W. Striley. "Marijuana Use among Adults 50 years and Older in the 21st Century." *Gerontology and Geriatric Medicine* (2018). https://www.ncbi.nlm.nih.gov/pmc/articles/PMC6024284/.

Lotan I., T. A. Treves, et al. "Cannabis (Medical Marijuana) Treatment for Motor and Non-Motor Symptoms of Parkinson Disease: An Open-Label Observational Study." *Clinical Neuropharmacology* (2014). https://pubmed.ncbi.nlm.nih.gov/24614667/.

Low Dog, Tieroana, MD; D. Kiefer, MD; R. Johnson, and S. Foster. *National Geographic Guide to Medicinal Herbs: The World's Most Effective Healing Plants*. Washington, DC: National Geographic, 2011.

Lyons, Christopher J., and Anthony G. Robson. "Retinal Ganglion Cell Dysfunction in Regular Cannabis Users: Is the Evidence Strong Enough to Consider an Association?" *JAMA Opthalmology* (2018). https://www.ncbi.nlm.nih.gov/pubmed/29450258.

Mammen, George. "Association of Cannabis with Long-Term Clinical Symptoms in Anxiety and Mood Disorders: A Systematic Review of Prospective Studies." *Journal of Clinical Psychiatry* (2018). https://www.ncbi.nlm.nih.gov/pubmed/29877641.

Masataka, Nobuo. "Anxiolytic Effects of Repeated Cannabidiol Treatment in Teenagers with Social Anxiety Disorders." *Frontiers of Psychology* (2019). https://www.ncbi.nlm.nih.gov/pmc/articles/PMC6856203/.

Mayo Clinic Radio. "Medical Marijuana with Dr. Jon Ebbert." https://www.youtube.com/watch?v=I1vwGRXYy3c

Meier, Madeline H., et al. "Associations between Cannabis Use and Cardiometabolic Risk Factors: A Longitudinal Study of Men." *Psychosomatic Medicine* (2019). https://www.ncbi.nlm.nih.gov/pubmed/30589665.

Miller, Sally, et al. "Controlled-Deactivation CB1 Receptor Ligands as a Novel Strategy to Lower Intraocular Pressure." *Pharmaceuticals* (2018). https://pubmed.ncbi.nlm.nih.gov/29786643/.

Mindell, Earl, RPH, MH, PhD. *Healing with Hemp CBD Oil: A Simple Guide to Using Powerful and Proven Health Benefits of CBD*. Garden City Park, NY: Square One Publishers, 2018.

Mitchell, John, et al. "'I Use Weed for My ADHD': A Qualitative Analysis of Online Forum Discussions on Cannabis Use and ADHD." *PLOS ONE* (2016). https://www.ncbi.nlm.nih.gov/pubmed/27227537.

Mokrysz, C., et al. "Are IQ and Educational Outcomes in Teenagers Related to Their Cannabis Use? A Prospective Cohort Study." *Journal of Psychopharmacology* (2016). https://www.ncbi.nlm.nih.gov/pmc/articles/PMC4724860/.

Morena, Maria, et al. "Neurobiological Interactions between Stress and the Endocannabinoid System." *Neuropsychopharmacology* (2016). https://www.ncbi.nlm.nih.gov/pmc/articles/PMC4677118/.

Muller-Val, Kirstin R. "Delta 9-Tetrahydrocannabinol (THC) Is Effective in the Treatment of Tics in Tourette Syndrome: A 6-Week Randomized Trial." *Journal of Clinical Psychiatry* (2003). https://www.ncbi.nlm.nih.gov/pubmed/12716250.

Nagappan, Arulkumar, et al. "Role of Cannabinoid Receptor Type 1 in Insulin Resistance and Its Biological Implications." *International Journal of Molecular Sciences* (2019). https://www.ncbi.nlm.nih.gov/pmc/articles/PMC6540410/.

Olah, Attila, et al. "Targeting Cannabinoid Signaling in the Immune System: 'High'-ly Exciting Questions, Possibilities, and Challenges." *Frontiers in Immunology* (2017). https://www.ncbi.nlm.nih.gov/pmc/articles/PMC5686045/.

Panahi, Yunes, et al. "The Arguments for and against Cannabinoids Application in Glaucomatous Retinopathy." *Biomedicine and Pharmacotherapy* (2017). https://www.ncbi.nlm.nih.gov/pubmed/28027538.

Parolaro, Daniela. "The Endocannabinoid System and Psychiatric Disorders." *Experimental Neurology* (2010). https://www.ncbi.nlm.nih.gov/pubmed/20353783.

Perron, Brian, et al. "Use of Prescription Pain Medications among Medical Cannabis Patients: Comparisons of Pain Levels, Functioning, and Patterns of Alcohol and Other Drug Use." *Journal of Studies on Alcohol and Drugs* (2015). https://pubmed.ncbi.nlm.nih.gov/25978826/.

Pini, A. "The Role of Cannabinoids in Inflammatory Modulation of Allergic Respiratory Disorders, Inflammatory Pain, and Ischemic Stroke." *Current Drug Targets* (2012). https://www.ncbi.nlm.nih.gov/pubmed/22420307.

Polat, Nihat, et al. "Corneal Endothelial Changes in Long-Term Cannabinoid Users." *Cutaneous and Ocular Toxicology* (2018). https://www.ncbi.nlm.nih.gov/pubmed/28427301.

Poli, P., et al. "Medical Cannabis in Patients with Chronic Pain: Effect on Pain Relief, Pain Disability, and Psychological Aspects." *La Clinica Terepeutica* (2018). https://www.ncbi.nlm.nih.gov/pubmed/29938740.

Prud'homme, Melissa. "Cannabidiol as an Intervention for Addictive Behaviors: A Systematic Review of the Evidence." *Substance Abuse* (2015). https://www.ncbi.nlm.nih.gov/pmc/articles/PMC4444130/.

Rappaport, Tina, BFA, and S. Leonard-Johnson, RN, PhD. *CBD-Rich Hemp Oil: Cannabis Medicine Is Back.* Scotts Valley, CA: CreateSpace, 2014.

Reiss, C. "Cannabinoids and Viral Infections." *Pharmaceuticals* (2010). https://www.ncbi.nlm.nih.gov/pmc/articles/PMC2903762/.

Romero, Kristoffer. "Multiple Sclerosis, Cannabis, and Cognition: A Structural MRI Study." *Neuroimage: Clinical* (2015). https://www.ncbi.nlm.nih.gov/pubmed/26106538.

Rudroff, Thorsten. "Cannabidiol to Improve Mobility in People with Multiple Sclerosis." *Frontiers in Neurology* (2018). https://www.ncbi.nlm.nih.gov/pubmed/29623067.

Russo, Ethan. "The Pharmacological History of Cannabis." In R. Pertwee, ed., *Handbook of Cannabinoids.* Oxford: Oxford University Press, 2014.

Russo, Ethan. "Taming THC: Potential Cannabis Synergy and Phytocannabinoid-Terpenoid Entourage Effects." *British Journal of Pharmacology* (2011). https://www.ncbi.nlm.nih.gov/pmc/articles/PMC3165946/.

———. "Introduction to the Endocannabinoid System." *Phytecs* (2015). https://www.phytecs.com/wp-content/uploads/2015/02/IntroductionECS.pdf.

———. "Clinical Endocannabinoid Deficiency Reconsidered: Current Research Supports Theory in Migraine, Fibromyalgia, Irritable Bowel, and Other Treatment-Resistant Syndromes." *Cannabis Cannabinoid Research* (2016). https://www.ncbi.nlm.nih.gov/pubmed/28861491.

———. "Cannabis Therapeutics and the Future of Neurology." *Frontiers of Integrative Science* (2018). https://www.ncbi.nlm.nih.gov/pmc/articles/PMC6200872.

Russo E., and G. W. Guy. "A Tale of Two Cannabinoids: The Therapeutic Rationale for Combining Tetrahydrocannabinol and Cannabidiol." *Medical Hypotheses* (2006). https://www.theroc.us/researchlibrary/Russo_A%20tale%20of%20two%20cannabinoids.pdf.

Russo, Ethan, and Andrea G. Hohmann. "Role of Cannabinoids in Pain Management." In *Comprehensive Treatment of Chronic Pain by Medical, Interventional, and Behavioral Approaches.*, edited by T.R. Deer, M.S. Leong, A. Buvanendran, V. Gordin, P.S. Kim, S.J. Panchal, A.L. Ray. New York: Springer, 2013.

Sawyer, Kristi. "Intergenerational Transmission of Depression: Clinical Observations and Molecular Mechanisms." *Molecular Psychiatry* (2018). https://www.ncbi.nlm.nih.gov/pubmed/30283036.

Scherma, Maria. "New Perspectives on the Use of Cannabis in the Treatment of Psychiatric Disorders." *Medicines* (2018). https://www.ncbi.nlm.nih.gov/pmc/articles/PMC6313625/.

Schleider, Lihi Bar-Lev, Mechoulam, Raphael, et al. "Real-life Experience of Medical Cannabis Treatment in Autism: Analysis of Safety and Efficacy." *Scientific Reports* (2019). https://www.ncbi.nlm.nih.gov/pmc/articles/PMC6336869/.

Schwitzer, Thomas. "The Endocannabinoid System in the Retina: From Physiology to Practical and Therapeutic Applications." *Neural Plasticity* (2016). https://www.ncbi.nlm.nih.gov/pmc/articles/PMC4736597/.

Shalaby, Michael. "Stirring the Pot: Cannabinoids and Atopic Dermatitis." *Practical Dermatology* (2018). https://practicaldermatology.com/articles/2018-jan/stirring-the-pot-cannabinoids-and-atopic-dermatitis.

Shamloul, Ramy, and Anthony J. Bella. "Impact of Cannabis Use on Male Sexual Health." *Journal of Sexual Medicine* (2011). https://www.ncbi.nlm.nih.gov/pubmed/21269404.

Sharma, Manju, et al. "In Vitro Anticancer Activity of Plant-Derived Cannabidiol on Prostate Cancer Cell Lines." *Pharmacology and Pharmacy* (2014). https://file.scirp.org/Html/5-2500510_47691.htm.

Shealy, Norman. *The Illustrated Encyclopedia of Healing Remedies*. New York: Harper Element, 2002.

Stanley, C. "Is the Cardiovascular System a Therapeutic Target for Cannabidiol?" *British Journal of Clinical Pharmacology* (2013). https://www.ncbi.nlm.nih.gov/pmc/articles/PMC3579247/.

Stapel, Britta. "Second Generation Atypical Antipsychotics Olanzapine and Aripiprazole Reduce Expression and Secretion of Inflammatory Cytokines in Human Immune Cells." *Journal of Psychiatric Research* (2018). https://www.ncbi.nlm.nih.gov/pubmed/30216787.

Steenkamp, Maria, et al. "Marijuana and Other Cannabinoids As a Treatment for Posttraumatic Stress Disorder: A Literature Review." *Depression and Anxiety* (2017). https://www.ncbi.nlm.nih.gov/pubmed/28245077.

Sun, Andrew, and Michael Eisenberg. "Association between Marijuana Use and Sexual Frequency in the United States: A Population-Based Study." *Journal of Sexual Medicine* (2017). https://www.ncbi.nlm.nih.gov/pubmed/29110804.

Testa, Maria, et al. "Marijuana Use Episodes and Partner Intimacy Experiences: A Daily Report Study." *Cannabis* (2019). https://www.ncbi.nlm.nih.gov/pubmed/30923794.

Thapa, D. "The Cannabinoids Δ8THC, CBD, and HU-308 Act via Distinct Receptors to Reduce Corneal Pain and Inflammation." *Cannabis and Cannabinoid Research* (2018). https://www.ncbi.nlm.nih.gov/pmc/articles/PMC5812319/.

Tibirica, E. "The Multiple Functions of the Endocannabinoid System: A Focus on the Regulation of Food Intake." *Diabetology and Metabolic Syndrome* (2010). https://www.ncbi.nlm.nih.gov/pmc/articles/PMC2832623/.

Toth, Kinga Fanni. "Cannabinoid Signaling in the Skin: Therapeutic Potential of the "C(ut)annabinoid" System." *Molecule* (2019). https://www.ncbi.nlm.nih.gov/pmc/articles/PMC6429381/.

Trainor, David. "Severe Motor and Vocal Tics Controlled with Sativex." *Australas Psychiatry* (2016). https://www.ncbi.nlm.nih.gov/pubmed/27558217.

Turcotte, C. "Impact of Cannabis, Cannabinoids, and Endocannabinoids in the Lungs." *Frontiers of Pharmacology* (2016). https://www.ncbi.nlm.nih.gov/pmc/articles/PMC5023687/.

US Food and Drug Administration. "FDA Approves First Drug Comprised of an Active Ingredient Derived from Marijuana to Treat Rare, Severe Forms of Epilepsy." FDA News Release. June 25, 2018. https://www.fda.gov/newsevents/newsroom/pressannouncements/ucm611046.htm.

Walsh, Zach, et al. "Medical Cannabis and Mental Health: A Guided Systematic Review." *Clinical Psychology Review* (2017). https://www.ncbi.nlm.nih.gov/pubmed/27816801.

Wang, Z., et al. "Treatment with a Cannabinoid Receptor 2 Agonist Decreases Severity of Established Cystitis." *Journal of Urology* (2013). https://www.jurology.com/article/S0022-5347(13)05841-2/abstract.

Web MD. "Medical Marijuana: What Does It Treat?" https://www.webmd.com/pain-management/video/medical-marijuana-2016.

White, Linda B., Barbara H. Seeber, and Barbara Brownell Grogan. *500 Time-Tested Home Remedies and the Science Behind Them*. Beverly, MA: Fair Winds Press, 2013.

Wong, Banny. "Pharmacogenetic Trial of a Cannabinoid Agonist Shows Reduced Fasting Colonic Motility in Patients with Nonconstipated Irritable Bowel Syndrome." *Gasteroenterology* (2011). https://www.ncbi.nlm.nih.gov/pubmed/21803011.

Yadav V., et al. "Summary of Evidence-Based Guideline: Complementary and Alternative Medicine in Multiple Sclerosis: Report of the Guideline Development Subcommittee of the American Academy of Neurology." *Neurology* (2014). https://pubmed.ncbi.nlm.nih.gov/24663230/.

WEBSITES

Charlotte's Web
https://www.cwhemp.com

Dr. Mary Clifton
https://doctormaryclifton.com/

Dr. Mary Clifton's Cannabis and CBD Info
http://cbdandcannabisinfo.com/

Healthline
https://www.healthline.com

Leafly: Cannabis 101, Growing, Strains, Politics, Health, Lifestyle, Science, and Tech
https://www.leafly.com

Marijuana Business Daily
https://mjbizdaily.com

Mayo Clinic
https://www.mayoclinic.org

Medicine Hunter
http://www.medicinehunter.com

Medline Plus, US National Library of Medicine
https://medlineplus.gov/

Medical News Today
https://www.medicalnewstoday.com/

Mind Body Green
https://www.mindbodygreen.com

Ministry of Hemp
https://ministryofhemp.com

National Conference of State Legislatures on State Industrial Hemp Statutes
http://www.ncsl.org/research/agriculture-and-rural-development/stateindustrial-hemp-statutes.aspx

National Hemp Association
https://nationalhempassociation.org

National Institutes of Health Library of Medicine
https://www.nlm.nih.gov

National Institute on Drug Abuse: Advancing Addiction Science
https://www.drugabuse.gov

Naturally Recovering Autism
https://naturallyrecoveringautism.com

Project CBD: Medical Marijuana and Cannabinoid Science
https://www.projectcbd.org

US Food and Drug Administration
https://www.fda.gov

Web MD
https://www.webmd.com

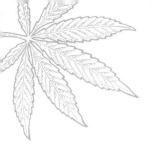

< **Acknowledgments** >

I am grateful to everyone in the NY cannabis community and beyond, especially but not limited to Vladamir Batista and the whole beautiful team at Happy Munkey, Michael O'Malley, Steve Bloom, Stu Zakim, Warren Bobrow, Chloe Villano, Jess Gonzalez, Shella Eckhouse, Oleg Mary Aces, Andrew Shattuck, Sherri Titkus, Gina Kranwinkel, Ashley Manning, and inspirations outside the cannabis community like Mary Agnes Antanopoulus, Dr. Tom O'Bryan, Dr. Christine Schaffner, Chris Winfeild, Jen Gottleib, JJ Virgin and Karl Krummanacher, Tim and Susan Bratton, Christopher Ulysses Walls, Matthew Schwartz, Brent Murphy, Brad Graham and Michael Dubanewicz, MD, Bonnie Goldstein, MD, Uma Dhanabalan, MD. For friends that helped me to create a path from insurance-reimbursed clinical practice to freedom and not forgetting to party along the way: Nancy Choi, Theresa Kadylak, Tanya Morgan, Bryce Johnson, Jeannie Kaufman, Chad Walkaden, and Jason Craigholm.

My SO Thom and kiddos Chelsea and Anna and cousin Jeannie Kaufman, sis Dawn Klemens for laughs and tears and love!

Mary Clifton MD

< 168 >

In my exciting and fulfilling journey to publish books that matter—on natural health and healing, I'd like to thank Jennifer Williams, Sterling executive editor, for her guidance and continuous font of ideas. She has paved the way for producing works on important and timely topics, such as *Cannabis for Health*. And her Sterling team—Renee Yewdaev, Shannon Plunkett, Igor Satanovsky, and Kevin Iwano—brought this beautiful product to fruition. Thanks to Laura Peet, who introduced me to Warren Bobrow in 2018. His book *Cannabis Cocktails, Mocktails, and Tonics* inspired a spirited conversation about the secrets of this little-known but powerful healing plant. I am grateful to Warren for immediately saying "Talk to Dr. Mary!" about bringing the story of healing cannabis to a wider audience. Dr. Mary Clifton's deep knowledge of and respect for the plant's medicinal qualities and her passionate concern for her patients has led us on the incomparable journey that puts this book in your hands. To writer Cathy Newman and photographer Lynn Johnson, former National Geographic colleagues whose beautiful coverage of medicinal cannabis instilled in me its vital healing potential. Always my thanks and love to Dan, Meredith, William, Caroline, and now Mirabelle. The future is bright.

< 169 >

< About the Authors >

MARY CLIFTON, MD, is a board-certified, licensed, internal medicine doctor based in Manhattan. She is a recognized expert in CBD and Cannabis and the founder of CBDandCannabisInfo.com and the highly respected professional certification course, The Cannabinoid Protocol. She provides specialized consultation on patient and provider education, telemedicine and cannabinoids, and has worked with several pharmaceutical, CBD, and cannabis corporations on areas of product development, speaking engagements, telemedicine, medical and scientific directorship in the US, Europe, Asia, and Africa.

Dr. Clifton is the bestselling author of *The Grass Is Greener: Medical Marijuana, THC & CBD OIL: Reversing Chronic Pain, Inflammation and Disease* and *Get Waisted*, as well as five companion cookbooks.

Her training tools teach healthcare providers and experts how to provide guidance and recommendations for their patients and clients.

Dr. Clifton is also a leading voice in telemedicine for bridging the gap in healthcare availability and affordability for acute care, long-term wellness and disability. She works in telemedical

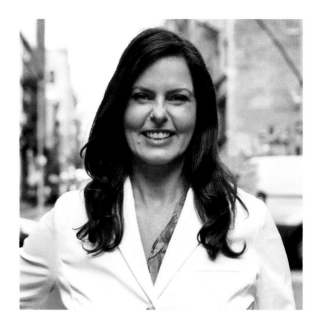

cannabinoid consultation and helps companies find telemedical solutions for their platforms and regularly sees patients from around the world on telemedicine platforms.

Dr. Clifton graduated magna cum laude from Michigan State University and attended medical school among the top primary care physicians at Michigan State University College of Human Medicine with high honor designations in internal medicine, family practice, pediatrics and obstetrics/gynecology. She was elected to join

< 170 >

the phi beta kappa honor society. She completed her internship and residency at MSU affiliated Spectrum Health in Grand Rapids, Michigan and served on the medical school's alumni board for 8 years. She has received research grants from BCBS of Michigan and is published in healthy lifestyle and diet.

Outside of the office, she lives in Manhattan and enjoys frequent travel, flavorful food, and rigorous yoga. She visits her two daughters frequently at their homes in Tennessee and Michigan.

You can follow her online:

www.TheCannabinoidProtocol.com

www.CBDandCannabisInfo.com

https://twitter.com/drmarymd

https://www.facebook.com/pg/DrMaryMd/

https://www.youtube.com/channel/
UCYWQ8H9L7RIIUkSNena8bCg

https://www.linkedin.com/in/marycliftonmd/detail/
recent-activity/

BARBARA BROWNELL GROGAN is former editor-in-chief of National Geographic Books and a certified health coach through New York's Institute for Integrative Nutrition. At National Geographic she developed the health and body line of reference books, with titles including Nature's Medicine and Medicinal Herbs. She has authored or co-authored five books on natural health and healing, including *500 Time-Tested Home Remedies and the Science Behind Them*, *Healing Herbs*, and the *CBD Handbook*.

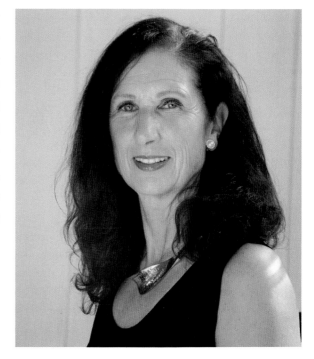

< Index >

Accidents, avoiding/reducing
  about: overview of, 44; types of
    accidents and statistics, 44
  current treatments, 44
  integrative tip, 46
  supporting research, 45–46
  Tony's story, 46
  why CBD/medical cannabis might
    be the answer, 44–45
ACDC strain, 33
Acne, 135–136
Adams, Roger, 9
Addiction and withdrawal, 46–49
  about: epidemic level of
    addiction and its impact,
    46–47
  current remedies, 47
  Dr. Hyla Cass on, 49
  integrative tip, 49
  Jennifer's story, 48
  supporting research, 48
  why CBD/medical cannabis might
    be the answer, 47–48
ADHD, 49–51
  about: perspective on impact and
    prevalence of, 49–50
  children using cannabis and, 59
  current remedies, 50
  integrative tip, 51
  Sondra's story, 51
  supporting research, 51
  why CBD/medical cannabis might
    be the answer, 50–51

Administering cannabis, 26–31
  about: portable vaporizers for,
    73; respiratory consequences of
    inhaling smoke, 79
  cannabis pipe for, 28–29
  edibles (foods, drinks, candy,
    lozenges), 31
  flower/bud option, trimming and
    care, 27–28
  one-hitter for, 30
  rolling papers for, 30–31
  tinctures, 31
  vape pen for, 26–27
  water pipe for, 29–30
ALS (amyotrophic lateral sclerosis),
  51–53
  about: background and reality of,
    51–52
  Alex's story, 53
  current remedies, 52
  integrative tip, 53
  supporting research, 53
  why CBD/medical cannabis might
    be the answer, 52
Amnesia Haze strain, 4
Analgesic cannabinoids, viii, 43. *See
also* Pain (acute and chronic); THC
(tetrahydrocannabinol)
Anandamide, 5, 11, 51, 83, 96, 127,
  130, 133
Anti-inflammatory cannabinoids,
  viii, 43
Anti-insomnia cannabinoid, 43

Antibacterial cannabinoids, viii, 43
Antidiabetic cannabinoid, 43
Antiemetic cannabinoids, 43
Antiepileptic cannabinoids, viii, 43
Antifungal cannabinoid, viii
Antimicrobial cannabinoid, 43
Antiproliferative cannabinoids, 43
Antispasmodic cannabinoids, 43
Antispasmodic treatments, 78
Anxiety, 53–56. *See also* Depression;
  Psychological conditions
  about: chronic, leading to
    problems, 22; diffuser blends
    for, 56; types/ranges of severity
    and effects of, 53–54
  current remedies, 54
  integrative tip, 56
  Steve's story, 56
  supporting research, 55
  why CBD/medical cannabis might
    be the answer, 54–55
Anxiolytic cannabinoids, 43
Appetite, controlling, 142, 143
Appetite, stimulating, viii, 39, 52, 58,
  79, 144
Armstrong, Louis, 12
Asthma. *See* Lung disease
Autism spectrum disorder (ASD),
  57–60
  about: spectrum and severity of,
    57
  Charlotte's story, 60
  children using cannabis and, 59

< 172 >

current remedies, 57–58
Dr. Elisa Song and, 60
integrative tip, 60
note from Dr. Mary, 59
supporting research, 59
why CBD/medical cannabis might
be the answer, 58–59
Autoimmune response/disease. *See*
Immune system health

Bipolar disorder. *See* Psychological
conditions
Blue Dream strain, 4
Blue Zones (heart-healthy places), 93
Bone stimulant cannabinoids, 43
Brain health, 61–66
about: perspectives on, 61–62;
watching TV and, 66
current remedies, 62–64
dementia, Alzheimer's and, 61, 62,
63, 65, 77, 102, 125, 127
Dr. Christine Schaffner and, 65
Ellie's story, 65
integrative tip, 66
stroke and, 61–62, 63, 64, 65, 88,
92, 114, 116
supporting research, 64–65
why CBD/medical cannabis might
be the answer, 63–64
Bratton, Susan, 107
Breathing exercise, 131, 139
Bubba Kush strain, 4
Buettner, Dan, 93

Cabeca, Dr. Anna, 149
Cancer and chemotherapy, 66–70.
See also Elder care and end of life
about: anticancer properties
of cabbage, 76–77;
antiproliferative cannabinoids
for, 43; chemotherapy,
cryoablation, and radiation
therapy, 67, 80; start of cancer,
66; types, impact, and statistics,
66–67

current treatments, 67, 78
integrative tip, 70
Melanie's story, 70
side effects reduced, 68–69
supporting research, 68–69
why CBD/medical cannabis might
be the answer, 67–68
Cannabichromene. *See* CBC
Cannabidiol. *See* CBD
Cannabidivarin (CBDV), 43
Cannabinoid receptors
about: overview of, viii–ix
diet and, 22
ECS and how they function, 3–5,
10–11
exercise and, 23
health conditions and (*See specific
conditions*)
sleep and, 23
stress management and, 23
Cannabinoids
ECS and, 2–5
helping with specific maladies
(*See specific conditions*)
how they work in the body, 3
potential health benefits by type
(charts), viii, 43
synthetic, 5
Cannabinol. *See* CBN
Cannabis
about: what it is, 2
author's (Dr. Mary's) personal
journey, ix–xi
detox and cleansing methods,
15–16
history of, vii–viii
Israeli research, 9–10, 45, 58, 96
legal considerations (*See* Legality
of cannabis)
medical use (*See* Healing with
cannabis; Medical marijuana)
in praise of, 1
proper care and trimming, 27–28
spirituality and, viii
stems and seeds, 28

word origin, vii
workplace and, 13–16
Cannabis sativa indica (recreational
marijuana), 2
Cannabis sativa (marijuana), 2
Cannabis sativa sativa (hemp), 2
Cass, Hyla, MD, 49
CBC (cannabichromene), viii,
10–11, 43
CBCA, viii
CBD (cannabidiol)
body's naturally occurring CBD, 5
cannabis strains and, 36–37, 38, 40
dosing and, 41
ECS and, 2–3
first research on, 9
health conditions and (*See specific
conditions*)
hemp characteristics and, 8
intoxication, testing and, 16
legality status, 12–13, 17
medicine today and, 9–11
potential health benefits, 43
testing for, workplace and, 13–16
THC vs., 9, 14
CBDA (cannabidiolic acid), viii, 10, 43
CBDV (cannabidivarin), 43
CBG (cannabigerol), viii, 43
CBGA, viii
CBN (cannabinol), viii, 28, 38, 43
Celiac disease. *See* Immune system
health
Charlotte's Web, 11. *See also* Figi,
Charlotte
Chemdawg strain, 34
Chernobyl strain, 34
Cherry AK strain, 4
Cherry Pie. *See* Harlequin strain
Children, cannabis and, 59, 84
Choosing cannabis. *See* Dispensaries;
specific strains; Strains of cannabis
Cleansing cannabis from your
system, 15–16
Crimea Blue strain, 34
Crystal Coma strain, 34

Cytokines
    cannabinoids and regulation of,
      95, 97, 100, 113
    immune response and, 93–94, 95
    influenza (flu) and, 99, 100
    Lyme disease and, 113

Death, old age and. *See* Elder care
  and end of life
Death Star strain, 34–35
Decarboxylation, 10
Delta 8-THC, viii
Delta 9-THC, viii
Depression, 70–73. *See also* Anxiety;
  Psychological conditions
    about: debilitating effect of, 70;
      long term effects, 22
    current remedies, 70, 71
    integrative tip, 73
    note from Dr. Mary, 72
    Oleg MaryAces on, 72, 73
    strain selection and
      administration for, 72
    supporting research, 72
    why CBD/medical cannabis might
      be the answer, 71–72
Detox and cleansing methods, 15–16
Diabetes. *See also* Metabolic
  syndrome
    diet and, 22
    eye health and, 85
    heart health and, 90, 92, 93
    inflammation and, 97
    neuropathic pain and, 121
    Terrence's story, 116
Diet
    anti-inflammatory, 98
    anticancer properties of cabbage,
      76–77
    balanced, ECS and, 22
    eating garnish on your plate, 125
    edible cannabis, 31
    salad and weight management, 144
    salt quality and virtues, 117
    spicy food benefits, 84–85

Diffuser blends, for anxiety, 56
Digestive health, 73–77. *See also*
  Nausea and vomiting
    about: intestinal anti-prokinetic
      cannabinoid, 43; prevalence and
      symptoms of GERD, IBS, and
      autoimmune IBDs, 73–74
    cabbage for, 76–77
    current remedies, 74–75
    Dr. Tom O'Bryan on, 76
    high-antioxidant foods/
      supplements, 128
    integrative tip, 76–77
    Samuel's story, 76
    supporting research, 75–76
    warm chicken soup for the flu, 101
    why CBD/medical cannabis might
      be the answer, 75
Dispensaries, 25–31
    administration options, 26–31
    choosing products/considerations,
      25–26
    dosing and, 41, 84
    menu of options at, 27
    quality of product, 28
    specific strains and their
      characteristics/effects (*See*
      Strains of cannabis)
    top-shelf buds, 28
Dosing, 41, 84
Dr. Grinspoon strain, 35
Dravet syndrome. *See* Epilepsy and
  seizures
Durban Poison strain, 35

Eckel, Dr. Greg, 127
Eczema, 134, 135, 136
Edibles (foods, drinks, candy,
  lozenges), 31
Elder care and end of life, 77–80. *See
also specific health conditions*
    about: perspectives on, 77
    avoiding falls, 80
    current treatments, 77–78
    integrative tip, 80

Jay's story, 80
    pain management, 77, 78, 79, 80
    supporting research, 79–80
    why CBD/medical cannabis might
      be the answer, 78–79
Endocannabinoid system (ECS)
    cannabinoid receptors and,
      viii–ix, 3 (*See also* Cannabinoid
      receptors)
    definition and function, 2–3
    inner cannabinoids and, 2, 3
    outer cannabinoids interacting
      with, 2–3
Endometriosis, 145, 146–147
Epilepsy and seizures, 80–85
    about: antiepileptic cannabinoids,
      viii, 43; causes and statistics,
      80–81; randomized trials on,
      82–83; syndromes associated
      with, 9, 80, 81, 82, 83; working
      closely with professionals, 84
    current remedies, 81–82
    Eleesha's story, 84
    integrative tip, 84–85
    note from Dr. Mary, 84
    strains and products
      considerations, 84
    supporting research, 83
    why CBD/medical cannabis might
      be the answer, 82–83
Erectile dysfunction. *See* Intimacy
  and fertility
Essential oils, for anxiety, 56
Euphoria strain, 35
Ewars, Dr. Keesha, 131
Exercise
    benefits of doing squats, 110–111
    brain health and, 62–63
    depression and, 73
    ECS and, 23
    psychological conditions and, 134
    replacing sedentary time with, 134
    skin health and, 134
Eye health, 85–87
    about: disease types and causes, 85

current remedies, 85–86
integrative tip, 87
Sally's story, 87
supporting research, 86–87
why CBD/medical cannabis might
   be the answer, 86

Fertility. *See* Intimacy and fertility
Figi, Charlotte, 11, 80, 82
Flower, cannabis, 27–28
Flu. *See* Influenza
Food. *See* Diet
Franklin, Benjamin, on hemp, 1

G-13, 35–36
GERD. *See* Digestive health
Ghost strain, 36
Girl Scout Cookie strain, 4, 36
Glossary of terms, 151–156
Godfather OG strain, 36
Grapes strain, 36
Green Crack strain, 4
Green Nurse Radio Show, 5

Harlequin strain, 36–37, 72
Hartridge, Caroline, DO, 144
Haze strain, 37
Headache and migraine, 87–90
   about: grounding yourself and,
      90; headache defined, 87;
      primary and secondary headache
      types/causes, 87–88; stress and,
      88 (*See also* Stress)
   current treatments, 88
   integrative tip, 90
   Kristine's story, 90
   supporting research, 89
   why CBD/medical cannabis might
      be the answer, 88–89
Headband strain, 4, 37
Healing with cannabis. *See also*
   Medical marijuana; *specific health
   conditions*
      balanced diet and, 22
      exercise and, 23

five roots of illness and, 21–22
general benefits by type of
   cannabinoid, viii, 43
history of, vii–viii, 7–9
pillars of integrative nutrition and
   ECS tone, 22–23
strain selection, 72
Heart health and disease, 90–93
   about: Blue Zones (heart-healthy
      places), 93; "broken heart"
      and death from, 90; causes of
      disease, 90–91
   current treatments, 91
   integrative tip, 93
   Pat's story, 93
   supporting research, 92–93
   why CBD/medical cannabis
      might be the answer, 91–92
Hemp, products and
   characteristics, 8
Herojuana strain, 4
Hibiscus tea, 87
History of cannabis, vii–viii, 7–9, 11–13
Hybrid strains, characteristics and
   examples, 4

IBS. *See* Digestive health
Immune system health, 93–96
   about: autoimmune response,
      94; celiac disease, 96; overview
      of immune system and
      imbalances of, 93–94; tongue
      care/health and, 96
   current remedies, 94–95
   integrative tip, 96
   Lewis's story, 96
   supporting research, 95–96
   why CBD/medical cannabis might
      be the answer, 95
Indica strains, characteristics and
   examples, 4
Inflammation, 96–98
   about: autoimmune diseases and,
      96; chronic, leading to problems,
      21, 96–97; immune response

and, 96 (*See also* Immune system
   health)
current treatments, 97
integrative tip, 98
Martin's story, 98
supporting research, 97–98
why CBD/medical cannabis might
   be the answer, 97
Influenza, 98–101
   about: pandemics, 99; symptoms,
      severity, contagiousness, 98–99;
      warm chicken soup for, 101
   current treatments, 99–100
   integrative tip, 101
   Shawn's story, 101
   supporting research, 100–101
   why CBD/medical cannabis might
      be the answer, 100
Insomnia, 101–103
   about: prevalence of, 101; risks of,
      101, 149; tip for falling asleep,
      103
   current remedies, 101–102
   integrative tip, 103
   Seymour's story, 103
   supporting research, 102–103
   why CBD/medical cannabis might
      be the answer, 102
   women's health and, 149
Integrative tips. *See specific health
   conditions*
Intimacy and fertility, 103–107
   about: aging and sex, 104;
      honoring your most important
      relationships, 107; importance
      of intimacy, 103; kinds of
      intimacy, 103; ups and downs
      and challenges of intimacy,
      103–104
   current treatments, 104–105
   integrative tip, 107
   supporting research, 106–107
   Susan Bratton's teachings, 107
   why CBD/medical cannabis might
      be the answer, 105–106

Jack Herer strain, 37

Kosher Kush strain, 37–38

Labels, what to look for when buying
cannabis, 25–26
Lavender strain, 38
Lee, Robert E., 1, 7
Legality of cannabis, 11–13
advocate Dr. David L Nathan
on, 19
benefits of/reasons for
legalization, 17–19
criminalization downsides, 8, 18
history of, 7–9, 11–13
move toward legalization,
16–19
recreational use, 12
testing cannabis use and, 13–16
workplace and, 13–16
worldwide, 17
Lennox-Gastaut syndrome. See
Epilepsy and seizures
Libido. See Intimacy and fertility
Lou Gehrig's disease. See ALS
(amyotrophic lateral sclerosis)
Lung disease, 107–111
about: asthma, 108–109,
110; benefits of doing squats,
110–111; bronchitis, 108,
109, 110; impact of, 107–108;
pulmonary fibrosis, 108, 109;
current treatments, 108–109
Debra's story, 110
integrative tip, 110–111
supporting research, 109–110
why CBD/medical cannabis might
be the answer, 109
Lyme disease, 111–113
about, 111–112; pulling tick from
skin, 113; symptoms, 111; tick
bites and, 111, 112
Charles's story, 113
current treatments, 112
integrative mandatory tip, 113

supporting research, 112–113
why CBD/medical cannabis might
be the answer, 112

Manic depression. See Psychological
conditions
Marijuana, products and
characteristics, 8. See also Strains
of cannabis
MaryAces, Oleg, 72, 73
Mazar strain, 38
Mechoulam, Dr. Raphael, 3, 9–10, 58
Medical marijuana
history of, 7–9
legal questions, 11–13
today and future of, 9–11
Medicine Man strain, 38
Menopause, 81, 105, 145, 146, 148,
149. See also Women's health
Metabolic syndrome, 114–117
about: age adding to
susceptibility, 114; blood tests
showing signs of, 114; defined,
114; overweight/obesity
triggering, 114; salt quality and
virtues, 117; symptoms setting
stage for, 114
current treatments, 114–115
integrative tip, 117
supporting research, 115–116
Terrence's story, 116
why CBD/medical cannabis might
be the answer, 115
Migraine. See Headache and
migraine
Mindset, putting on daily, 141
Multiple sclerosis (MS), 117–120
about: description and symptoms,
117; integrative practices
supporting pharmaceutical
regimen, 119; working closely
with professionals, 120
current remedies, 117–118
Devon's story, 119
integrative tip, 119

note from Dr. Mary, 120
strains and products
considerations, 119
supporting research, 119
why CBD/medical cannabis might
be the answer, 118

Nathan, David L., MD, DFAPA, 19
Nausea and vomiting. See also
Digestive health
cannabis relieving, 10, 68, 75, 79,
80, 95, 147
historical use of cannabis, viii, 1
immune system (cytokines)
causing, 94
Nausea-reducing cannabinoids, 43
Neuropathic pain. See Pain (acute
and chronic)
Neuroprotective cannabinoids, 43
Nonpsychoactive cannabinoids, 43
Northern Lights strain, 4
Nurses, handbook for, 5
NYC Diesel strain, 38

O'Bryan, Dr. Tom, 76
OG Kush strain (and hybrids), (36),
(37), 38–39
One-hitter, 30
O'Shaughnessy, William Brooke, 1

Pain (acute and chronic), 120–125.
See also Elder care and end of life;
Headache and migraine; Multiple
sclerosis (MS)
about: acute pain defined, 120;
chronic pain defined, 120–121;
chronic pain syndromes, 121;
older adults and, 121; personal
nature of pain and treatment,
120, 121
Carl's story, 124
current treatments to consider,
121–123
Dr. Michele Ross's expertise, 125
integrative tip, 125

neuropathic pain, 98, 117, 121, 122, 123–124

strains and products considerations, 124

why CBD/medical cannabis might be the answer/supporting research, 123–124

Papers, rolling, 30–31

Parkinson's disease, 125–128

about: high-antioxidant foods/supplements helping with, 128; symptoms and what scientists know, 125

current treatments, 125–126

Dr. Greg Eckel and, 127

integrative tip, 128

Neely's story, 127

supporting research, 126–127

why CBD/medical cannabis might be the answer, 126

Phytocannabinoids, 5, 10–11. See also CBD; THC

Piffard, Dr. Henry Granger, 135

Pineapple Express, 4

Pipes

cannabis, 28–29

water, 29–30

Plaque

brain health and, 61–62, 65

CBD, cannabinoids and, 65, 92, 116, 135, 136

heart disease and, 90–91, 92

metabolic syndrome and, 114, 116

skin conditions and, 134, 135, 136

PMS. See Women's health

Post-traumatic stress disorder (PTSD), 128–131

about: brain function and, 128; breathing exercise to relax body, 131, 139; hyperarousal syndrome and, 128–129; symptoms of, 128

current remedies, 129

Dr. Keesha Ewars and, 131

integrative tip, 131

supporting research, 130

Trevor's story, 130

why CBD/medical cannabis might be the answer, 129–130

Psoriasis, 134, 135–136

Psychoactive cannabinoids, 43

Psychological conditions, 131–134. See also Anxiety; Depression

about: bipolar disorder, 131, 132–133; schizophrenia, 131–132, 133

Agnes's story, 133

current remedies, 132

integrative tip, 134

mania precaution for synthetic THC, 132–133

supporting research, 133

why CBD/medical cannabis might be the answer, 132–133

Pulmonary fibrosis. See Lung disease

Purple Kush strain, 39

Red Congo/Congolese strain, 39

Rolling papers, 30–31

Romulan strain, 39

Ross, Michele, PhD, 125

Salt, quality and virtues, 117

Sativa strains, characteristics and examples, 4

Schaffner, Dr. Christine, 65

Schizophrenia. See Psychological conditions

Seasoning food heavily, benefits, 84–85

Seizures. See Epilepsy and seizures

Sex and sex drive. See Intimacy and fertility

Skin conditions, 134–136

about: overview of types/causes/symptoms, 134–135

acne, 135–136

atopic dermatitis (eczema), 134, 135, 136

current remedies, 135

Dani's story, 136

integrative tip, 136

psoriasis, 134, 135–136

supporting research, 136

why CBD/medical cannabis might be the answer, 135–136

Skunk strain, 39

Skywalker OG strain, 4

Sleep

difficulties (See Insomnia)

downsides of deprivation, 21, 149

ECS contributions, 23

quality, benefits of, 23

Socialization, ECS and, 23

Song, Elisa, MD, 60

Sour Diesel strain, 4. See also NYC Diesel

Spasticity. See ALS (amyotrophic lateral sclerosis); Multiple sclerosis (MS)

Spices and herbs, 85

Spicy food, benefits, 84–85

Spirituality, ECS and, 23

Squats, benefits of, 110–111

Strains of cannabis

about: dosing and, 41; overview of selecting strains, 33; Sativa/Indica/hybrid characteristics and examples, 4; species and subspecies, 2

ACDC, 33

Charlotte's Web, 11

Chemdawg, 34

Chernobyl, 34

Crimea Blue, 34

Crystal Coma, 34

Death Star, 34–35

Dr. Grinspoon, 35

Durban Poison, 35

Euphoria, 35

G-13, 35–36

Ghost, 36

Girl Scout Cookie, 4, 36

Godfather OG, 36

Strains of cannabis (*cont.*)
  Grapes, 36
  Harlequin, 36–37, 72
  Haze, 37
  Headband, 4, 37
  Jack Herer, 37
  Kosher Kush, 37–38
  Lavender, 38
  Mazar, 38
  Medicine Man, 38
  NYC Diesel, 38
  OG Kush (*and hybrids*), (*36*), (*37*),
    38–39
  Purple Kush, 39
  Red Congo/Congolese, 39
  Romulan, 39
  Skunk, 39
  Sour Diesel, 4 (*See also* NYC
    Diesel strain)
  Sunset Sherbet, 39–40
  Tangie, 40
  Trainwreck, 40
  Wedding Cake, 40
Stress, 136–139. *See also* Post-
  traumatic stress disorder (PTSD)
  about: breathing exercise to
    relax body, 131, 139; chronic,
    leading to problems, 21;
    headaches and, 88; overview
    and effects of, 136–137
  Angela's story, 138
  current remedies, 137
  integrative tip, 138–139
  managing, ECS and, 23
  supporting research, 138
  why CBD/medical cannabis
    might be the answer, 138
Stroke. *See* Brain health
Sturge-Weber syndrome. *See* Epilepsy
  and seizures
Stuttering. *See* Tics and Tourette
  syndrome (TS)/stuttering
Sulak, Dr. Dustin, 106–107
Sunset Sherbet strain, 39–40

Tangie strain, 40
Television, brain health and, 66
Testing for cannabis use, 13–16
Tetrahydrocannabinolic acid. *See*
  THCA
THC (tetrahydrocannabinol)
  amount in hemp, 8
  amount in marijuana, 8 (*See
    also specific strains of marijuana*)
  children, cannabis and, 59
  detox and cleansing methods,
    15–16
  dosing and, 41
  ECS and, 2–3
  enhancing body's repair
    functions, 5
  first research on, 9
  health conditions and (*See specific
    conditions*)
  legality status, 11–13, 16–19, 25
  marijuana characteristics and, 8
  medicine today and, 9–11
  percent in purchased products,
    25
  testing for, 13–15
THCA (tetrahydrocannabinolic acid),
  viii, 10, 43
THCV, viii
Tics and Tourette syndrome (TS)/
  stuttering, 139–141
  about: daily mindset and, 141;
    symptoms and origins/causes,
    139
  current remedies, 139–140
  integrative tip, 141
  Rennie's story, 141
  why CBD/medical cannabis
    might be the answer/
    supporting research,
    140–141
Tinctures, 31
Tongue, caring for, 96
Tourette syndrome. *See* Tics and
  Tourette syndrome (TS)/stuttering

Trainwreck strain, 40
Tutkus, Sherri, 5
2-arachidonoylglycerol, 5, 51, 72

Vape pen, 26–27
Vaporizers, portable, 73
Vasoconstriction cannabinoid, 43
Vomiting. *See* Nausea and vomiting

Water pipe, 29–30
Wedding Cake strain, 40
Weight management, 141–144. *See
  also* Metabolic syndrome
  about: balance in life and, 142;
    perspective on, 141–142;
    process of weight gain/loss, 142;
    salad and, 144
  current treatments, 142
  David's story, 144
  Dr. Caroline Hartridge and, 144
  integrative tip, 144
  supporting research, 143–144
  why CBD/medical cannabis might
    be the answer, 142–143
White Rhino. *See* Medicine Man
  strain
Women's health, 145–149
  about: overview of issues, 145;
    sleep and, 149
  current treatments, 146
  Dr. Anna Cabeca and, 149
  endometriosis and, 145, 146–147
  integrative tip, 149
  Meeghan's story, 148
  menopause and, 81, 105, 145, 146,
    148, 149
  PMS and, 145, 146
  supporting research, 147–148
  why CBD/medical cannabis might
    be the answer, 146–147
Workplace, cannabis use/testing,
  13–16

< **Photo Credits** >

< 179 >

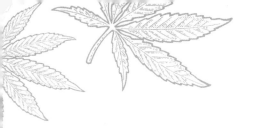

< **Other Books in the Series** >

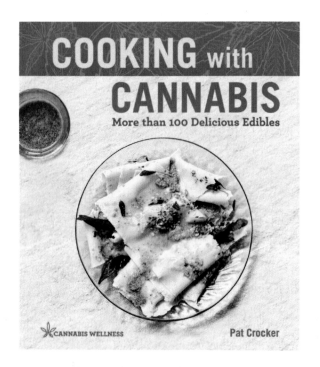

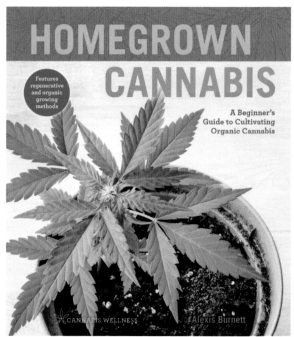

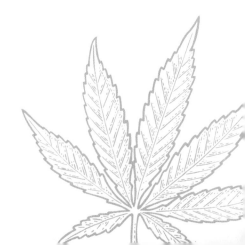